Embracing Change

Trusting God Through the Transitions of Life

JUST DAWN LOVE

FOREWORD BY PASTOR NATASHA ROCKMORE

Published by Beyond the Book Media

Beyond The Book Media, LLC

Atlanta. GA

www.beyondthebookmedia.com

ISBN: 978-1-953788-95-5

Title: Embracing Change: Trusting God through Life's Transitions

Description: First edition. | [Atlanta]: [Beyond the Book Media], 2023.

Subjects: BISAC: SELF-HELP / Personal Growth

Printed in ["the United States of America"]

Interior layout by Beyond The Book Media All rights reserved.

Embracing Change

Trusting God Through the Transitions of Life

JUST DAWN LOVE

FOREWORD BY PASTOR NATASHA ROCKMORE

DEDICATION

To my three pillars of strength, Reginald II, Ryan, and Randall: You are my inspiration and my heart's most profound joys. To my parents, who laid the foundation of love, faith, and perseverance upon which I stand. And to Solomon, the unexpected light on my journey, guiding me through the chapters of life with unwavering support. This book is a testament to the love and lessons you've all instilled in me. With all my love and gratitude.

FOREWORD

There is such an authentic expression with Dawn Love. Her life of integrity is full of inspiration. I truly believe that as you turn the pages or scroll the pages on your electronic device, or perhaps listen as you travel this road called life, you will be invigorated to see every trial, challenge, struggle, etc., as an investment to evolve. The mask of shame will be shaped into a canvas of beauty.

As I read, a soft smile came across my face. Why? You will soon find out. Through every word, you will hear not just another woman telling her secrets, but rather a woman who has to have trust in her GOD. I encourage you not to rush through the pages but to allow them to simmer in your heart and mind, knowing and understanding that if Dawn can stand after all she has endured, you can also stand on the shoulders of her story and not collapse.

Dawn, congratulations to you! This is just the beginning! I am grateful to be a part of the revealing of your journey. Great grace to you!

NaTasha S. Rockmore

TABLE OF CONTENTS

ACKNOWLEDGMENTS

First and foremost, my deepest gratitude goes to God. In times when my strength wavered, it was His unyielding power that carried me through.

To my beloved children, who have been the driving force behind every word and every lesson this book encompasses. To my parents, whose wisdom and guidance have been my north star. And to Solomon, whose presence has been nothing short of a blessing, making this journey richer and more meaningful.

A heartfelt thank you to my besties, LaSuria and Linnetia, and my dear Betty. Our talks, your unwavering faith in me, and the encouragement you've generously showered upon me have been the anchor I needed to bring this book to life.

And to every individual finding themselves amidst a life transition, this book is for you. It is a testament to resilience, hope, and the promise of a new dawn. May you find solace and strength in these pages, just as I have in living through and penning down these experiences."

INTRODUCTION

Welcome, dear reader, to the pages of "Embracing Change: Trusting God Through the Transitions of Life." This book is the embodiment of my journey, my heart, and the wisdom I have gathered along the way. My name is inscribed on the cover, but it is the experiences enclosed within that truly define me as an author.

From the moment I took my first breath, my journey has been marked by an unending series of transitions. Now I comprehend why God entrusted me with this platform–Transitions. As a Christian woman, my path to authorship was neither linear nor easy. It was forged from numerous transitions, each one molding, defining, and ultimately motivating me to write this book. I have encountered a wide range of adversities–from abortion, bankruptcy, and mental health challenges to the terrifying experience of rape, the burdensome weight of unforgiveness and jealousy, foreclosure, and the raw, deep piercing pain of divorce. Additionally, I took on the role of a single mother to three boys–a journey in itself. I have endured the most daunting storms life could muster and, through it all, found a way to emerge stronger.

The scars etched into my soul by these experiences have qualified me in a way that no degree or certification could. They have taught me to find strength in vulnerability, to see every challenge as a stepping stone, and to trust in God's divine plan through the turmoil. It is these lessons that I bring forth in this book, with the hope that they can guide you through your own transitions.

"Embracing Change: Trusting God Through the Transitions of Life" is more than just a recounting of my experiences. It is a shared journey through the peaks and valleys of life, a journey I hope will foster resilience and fortitude within you. Each chapter is a testament to the transformative power of faith, offering tools and strategies to navigate life's transitions with grace, courage, and unshakable trust in God.

By journeying through these pages, you will learn to view transitions not as insurmountable obstacles but as opportunities for growth and personal evolution. You will find strategies for dealing with emotional upheaval, practical tips for rebuilding your life after a major setback, and, most importantly, you will discover the power of forgiveness and letting go.

The lessons gleaned from my experiences are not sugar-coated truths or quick fixes. They are real, raw, and deeply personal, grounded in empathy, compassion, and understanding. As you read this book, know you are not alone in your struggles. I have been where you are, I have felt what you feel, and I am a testament to the fact that there is light at the end of the darkest tunnel.

This book is your guide, your friend, and your companion through life's tumultuous transitions. I hope that as you turn each page, you will find not just my story but pieces of your own. By the end of this journey, you will emerge stronger, wiser, and filled with an invincible faith that will guide you through any storm.

I encourage you to embark on this journey with me. Despite the pain, confusion, and upheaval, remember that you are not alone and that each step you take is a step toward healing, growth, and a brighter future. Embrace the change, trust in God, and remember: the only constant in life is transition itself. Let's navigate it together. Welcome to "Embracing Change: Trusting God Through the Transitions of Life."

1 CHANGE'S UNYIELDING TIDE: UNPACKING LIFE'S INEVITABILITIES

~Understanding Transitions~

Do you remember the feeling of outgrowing a beloved pair of shoes from childhood? Those shoes held memories of first steps, backyard adventures, and countless games of catch. But as the days turned to months and then years, your feet began to grow, and suddenly, those shoes felt tight. Uncomfortable. Restricting. A change was inevitable.

Life's transitions are much like outgrowing those cherished shoes. There are times when what once felt comfortable becomes confining, pushing us into unknown territories. Each of us, at some point in our lives, encounter moments when the familiar landscape shifts, be it due to a job change, moving to a new city, or undergoing personal transformations. Such moments might make us feel lost, uncertain, or even scared.

This chapter aims to shed light on the nature of life's transitions. It's here that we'll demystify the difference between mere change—a simple alteration of the status quo—and a genuine transition, which is a deeper, more intricate process of adaptation and growth. By understanding these processes, you'll find yourself better prepared, not just to cope but to thrive.

The journey of life is filled with numerous transitions, each offering its own set of challenges and lessons. Through this chapter, I hope to provide a clearer picture of these moments of change, making them more relatable and less daunting. Like that pair of shoes, it's essential to recognize when it's time to move on, to embrace new experiences, and to step confidently into the next phase of your journey. Let's walk this path together.

~The Nature of Life's Transitions: A Glimpse Through Naomi's Journey~

Following the theme of understanding transitions, it's clear that shifts and changes are inseparable from the rhythm of life itself. Just as seasons come and go and tides rise and fall, change is an undeniable principle governing our existence. The complexities of these life shifts can be overwhelming and differ in their effects and challenges, but they offer one unifying gift: the opportunity for transformation.

Delving into the annals of Biblical history, one finds an embodiment of life's transitions in the character of Naomi from the Book of Ruth. Naomi's journey was not a straightforward path of joy and contentment but one riddled with sharp turns of fate, intense loss, and profound transformation.

Her story begins in Bethlehem, where a severe famine prompted Naomi, her husband, and her two sons to migrate to Moab. In Moab, tragedy befell her. She lost her husband and later both her sons, rendering her not just a widow but also childless—a vulnerable status in those times. Naomi's life had taken an unforeseen transition from stability in Bethlehem to despair in Moab.

Yet, it is the nature of life's transitions to offer choices, even amidst despair. Facing her grief, Naomi made the pivotal decision to return to Bethlehem, urging her two daughters-in-law, Orpah and Ruth, to stay in Moab and rebuild their lives. While Orpah chose the comfort of the familiar, Ruth clung to Naomi, uttering the immortal words, "Where you go, I will go; where you lodge, I will lodge; your people shall be my people, and your God my God" (Ruth 1:16).

This decision marked another transition, not just in location but in the very dynamics of Naomi's life. Ruth's loyalty and commitment brought a rejuvenated sense of purpose and hope to Naomi's life, culminating in Ruth marrying Boaz, a relative of Naomi, ensuring security and lineage continuation.

Naomi's journey—from Bethlehem to Moab and back, from joy to despair to hope—is a powerful testament to the nature of life's transitions. Each change, each decision, bore consequences that reshaped her destiny. Her narrative is a poignant reminder that while transitions can be challenging, harrowing even, they also carry the seeds of renewal and growth.

Drawing from Naomi's story, it's evident that life's transitions are neither entirely good nor bad. They are complex webs of events that shape, mold, and transform us. Just as Naomi emerged from her trials with renewed hope, our transitions, too, hold the potential for profound personal evolution.

In the face of life's inevitable changes, the scripture from James 1:2-4 serves as a beacon: "Consider it pure joy, my brothers and sisters, whenever you face trials of many kinds, because you know that the testing of your faith produces perseverance." Much like Naomi, our faith, perseverance, and the choices we make during transitions can lead us to unexpected blessings and a deeper understanding of life's intricate design.

~Recognizing the Inevitability of Change: Life's Sole Constant~

Reflecting on the deep insights about life's transitions, one is naturally led to a foundational realization that underpins these changes: the certainty of change itself. Just as the sun reliably gives way to the moon and winter inevitably yields to spring, change is embedded in the very core of our existence.

If one were to ponder their personal experiences or observe the expansive panorama of the world, it becomes abundantly clear that life is in a perpetual state of flux. Seasons shift, civilizations rise and fall, and even the sturdiest mountains erode over time. Nothing remains static, and therein lies the beauty and challenge of existence.

One might argue, however, that recognizing the inevitability of change is a daunting realization. After all, humans inherently seek stability, safety, and predictability. Yet, it's this very quest for permanence in a world defined by transience that often leads to profound disquiet.

Drawing parallels with the narrative of Naomi, change was neither sought nor welcomed. She faced a series of unwelcomed changes, from displacement due to famine to the devastating loss of her loved ones. But Naomi's story didn't end in Moab; it was her acceptance of change, her recognition of its inevitability, that led her back to Bethlehem and into a new chapter of restoration and hope.

Similarly, our trials often stem not from change itself, but from our resistance to change, which often breeds suffering. In denying change, we are essentially denying the very nature of life. Embracing change doesn't demand passive acceptance but rather a proactive engagement with the ebbs and flows of existence.

This sentiment finds resonance in the teachings of ancient philosophers and sages. The Buddhists preach about the impermanence of life, emphasizing that understanding and accepting this truth is the path to enlightenment. Stoic philosophers, too, advocated for recognizing the unpredictability of life and finding tranquility in accepting what we cannot control.

Flowing from our exploration of life's transitions, recognizing the inevitability of change offers a deeper layer of understanding. It encourages us to move beyond mere acceptance of individual transitions to a broader acknowledgment of life's inherent unpredictability.

In doing so, we are equipped with a resilience that's not just reactive but proactive. We don't merely weather the storms; we learn to dance in the rain. We follow in the footsteps of Naomi, who found hope and renewal not despite change but because of it. For in the ever-changing theater of life, it's not the scenes that define our story but how we choose to navigate them.

~ The Nuances of Change and Transition: A Dance of External and Internal Dynamics~

As we dig a little deeper into the ever-changing landscape of our lives, we come to a subtle but important realization: change and transition aren't the same thing. Many of us use these words like they're interchangeable, but truly grasping the subtle differences between them can offer us some game-changing insights into who we are and who we're becoming, both personally and spiritually.

Change, in its essence, is external—a tangible shift in circumstances, environments, or situations. It's the departure of a loved one, the shifting of a job, or the movement from one city to another. These are observable, often measurable, alterations in the external world. This concept is reflected, though in different terms, in the Book of Isaiah, where it is written: "See, I am doing a new thing! Now it springs up; do you not perceive it?" (Isaiah 43:19). This verse reinforces the idea that change is an ever-present, divinely inspired facet of our lives, constantly unfolding in various ways around us and even being orchestrated by forces beyond our immediate understanding. It calls on us to recognize and embrace these shifts as part of our spiritual journey.

Transition is more about what's happening within us than around us. It's the personal journey that we go through and the internal work we do when faced with new circumstances. Let's think about when a close friend or a family member, someone you've spent countless hours with, suddenly has less time for you or perhaps moves on in some way. The change is clear: you're seeing less of each other, and the dynamic of your relationship shifts.

But the transition is what happens inside you after this. It's wrestling with feelings of loneliness, reassessing your self-worth outside of that friendship, and learning to invest time and emotion in new people or hobbies. It's realizing that your identity isn't tied to one person or relationship and rebuilding your inner strength and sense of self. This period of inner transformation, the transition, can be challenging and often requires more time and self-exploration than adjusting to the external aspects of the change. It's about redefining your beliefs about yourself and finding new ways to relate to your world.

Drawing inspiration from the words of the renowned Christian motivational speaker, Dr. Charles Stanley: "The circumstances of our lives are pieces of a larger scheme in the puzzle of life, and in His Perfect Wisdom, the pieces fit." This quote underscores the idea that while external changes (the pieces) shape our lives, it's our internal transitions that give them meaning and purpose, helping us discern the bigger picture.

Let's circle back to Naomi. Her life was marked by profound changes: famine, migration, and personal loss. Yet, the heart of her story isn't just about these changes but her transitions—the spiritual and emotional metamorphosis she underwent. Her journey from bitterness, as she even named herself "Mara," which means "bitter," to a renewed sense of hope and faith in God's plan, is a testament to the transformative power of transition.

To truly navigate life's unpredictable terrain, it's imperative to recognize and honor both change and transition. Changes might be inevitable, as previously reflected upon, but transitions are our intentional, mindful responses to these changes. They are where our spiritual growth is cultivated, where our character is refined, and where we find deeper alignment with God's purpose for our lives.

While the world around us continually shifts, presenting a kaleidoscope of changes, our inner world has the potential to transition, guiding us toward greater wisdom, resilience, and faith. Embracing change and transition ensures not just our survival but our blossoming in the beautiful, intricate garden of life.

2 BARING THE SOUL: THE UNEXPECTED POWER IN VULNERABILITY

~Vulnerability as Strength~

Picture this: a tiny seed buried beneath layers of soil. At first glance, it seems weak, insignificant, and easily crushed. Yet, with time, water, and sunlight, it pushes through the dirt, breaking open in the process. This rupture, though it may seem like a sign of fragility, is actually the seed's greatest strength— it allows it to grow, to sprout, and to eventually bloom into a magnificent flower or a towering tree.

Similarly, in our lives, there are moments when we might feel like that buried seed—trapped, overwhelmed, and fragile. Society often tells us to mask our true feelings, to put up a brave front, and to hide any sign of 'weakness.' But what if, much like that seed, our moments of vulnerability are not our weaknesses but our strengths?

In this chapter, we'll delve deep into the essence of vulnerability. We'll explore how showing our true selves, wounds and all, can lead to deeper connections, greater understanding, and a more authentic life experience. Together, we'll challenge the conventional views on vulnerability, seeking to embrace it as an avenue for growth, learning, and empowerment.

Through personal anecdotes and shared experiences, you'll see that the times you feel most vulnerable can also be the moments of your greatest strength. It's in these moments that you truly connect with yourself and others, and it's through these connections that you tap into the powerful, transformative energy of vulnerability. Let's embark on this journey of rediscovering and redefining strength.

~My Journey of Embracing Vulnerability: Strength Amidst the Storms of Life~

Life is like a painting, and we are all artists in our own right. One thing's for sure: things are always changing. For the longest time, I treated being vulnerable like it was a big blot of the wrong color on my life's artwork. It felt like a mistake, not something that made the picture more real or deep.

I remember when I was younger, I thought letting my guard down meant I was weak. At school, you were supposed to be tough; you couldn't let teasing or setbacks show they bothered you. And when I started working, it felt like I had to be even stronger, like any crack in my armor would make people think I wasn't good enough. So, I built this wall around me, thinking it made me invincible.

But life has a way of throwing curveballs at you. For me, it was my divorce. There were no dramatic courtroom showdowns or fights over who'd get what. Just two people, deeply hurt, dealing with their own pains and pasts, unable to fix what we once thought was unbreakable. We were broken and trying to navigate through the mess of feelings was tough. I was swirling in a storm of guilt, frustration, a sense of loss, and feeling more vulnerable than ever. It was like standing in the middle of a crowd with all my fears and failures on display.

It wasn't just about splitting up; it felt like I was tearing down everything I believed about myself. I wasn't just losing a marriage; I was losing a part of who I was. But here's the thing — it was during this rock-bottom moment that I began to see that vulnerability wasn't my weakness. It was the gateway to my deepest strength.

During one of these tumultuous days, a conversation with a dear friend offered a glimmer of clarity. As tears blurred my vision, I hesitated but decided to share my inner turmoil. Her response, punctuated by a compassionate embrace, was simple yet profound, "It's alright to hurt. Remember, even Jesus wept."

This biblical reference to John 11:35, the shortest verse in the Bible, reminded me that vulnerability is not a departure from strength but an embodiment of it.

It was then that I embarked on a transformative journey of embracing my vulnerability. Guided by Brené Brown's insightful words, "Vulnerability is not winning or losing; it's having the courage to show up and be seen when we have no control over the outcome," I began to open up about my feelings, fears, and hopes. This act of raw authenticity, while initially daunting, became my anchor. It paved the way for deeper connections, self-acceptance, and a profound understanding of God's purpose for me, even in times of pain.

In the grand spectrum of life, vulnerability, with its beautiful imperfections, holds a significant place. It's about our shared experiences as people, our deep need to feel connected with others, and the real strength that lives inside us. When we go through tough times, particularly huge life changes like going through a divorce, showing our vulnerable side isn't about giving up. Instead, it's like wearing a badge of bravery and strength, proving we can face challenges and keep going.

~ The Power of Openness and Authenticity: Emerging from Silence~

Life's symphony is a complex arrangement composed of various melodies and harmonies that dance to the rhythm of change. Amid this composition, some notes are more difficult to strike than others. For many, vulnerability is one such note, buried deep and often left untouched. However, I've realized that sometimes the most beautiful melodies arise when we summon the courage to play these very notes.

After the turbulent waves of divorce, I had a significant revelation: shielding myself from vulnerability wasn't fortifying me; it was stifling my true essence. And while the dissolution of my marriage had made me reevaluate many things, there was another part of my past that I had buried even deeper.

For 38 long years, a dark secret weighed heavily on my heart. A painful memory so shrouded in shame and fear that I had locked it away, hoping time would erode its edges. But some wounds, if left untreated, fester. It was the traumatic experience of sexual assault, a violation so profound that words fail to capture its entirety. I had been silenced, not just by society's stigmas but by my own internalized fears.

Then came a moment, much like a sudden break in stormy clouds, when a beam of understanding pierced through. If I had found strength in the vulnerability of sharing my post-divorce sentiments, perhaps there was power in opening up about this deeply personal trauma, too. Inspired by this newfound perspective, I took my first tentative steps toward authenticity and openness.

One day at work, I found myself immersed in a profound moment of courage. I decided it was time to call my mom and unveil the painful secret I had carried for so long about being sexually assaulted by a family member one summer in South Carolina. I was apprehensive, uncertain if she would be angry at me for what had occurred or frustrated because I had kept it to myself for 38 agonizing years. The reaction I received, however, was one of pure compassion, a response I hadn't anticipated.

Despite her understanding, a wave of anger soon washed over me, a mixture of self-blame and the haunting question of how such a thing could have been permitted to happen. The incident has left an indelible scar on my memory. Sharing my story was an uphill battle. In the beginning, the words hardly came out, caught in a chokehold of raw emotion and tears. But there was a transformative power in the retelling: with each occasion I spoke of it, the heavy shackles of shame started to loosen. My experience, which had felt like solitary confinement, slowly turned into a bridge, reaching out to others who had suffered in similar ways. It forged connections, a shared understanding, and a collective healing that made us all stronger together.

Scripture says in James 5:16, "Confess your sins to each other and pray for each other so that you may be healed." It's a testament to the healing power of openness. By speaking my truth, not only was I seeking healing, but I was also offering solace to others, reminding them they were not alone.

In embracing authenticity, I recognized its unparalleled power. My rape, though a harrowing experience, became a testament to resilience, survival, and the transformative power of vulnerability. Authenticity and openness didn't erase the pain, but they illuminated the path to healing and liberation.

The journey to wholeness is punctuated with moments of profound courage. In my narrative, the courage to be open and authentic about my rape after decades of silence stands as a beacon of hope. It's a poignant reminder that even in our most vulnerable truths, there lies an indomitable strength waiting to be discovered.

~Overcoming Societal Pressures to "Stay Strong": Embracing My Brokenness~

In the journey of life, filled with diverse experiences, society frequently nudges us to frame our narratives exclusively from the perspective of unwavering strength. Strength is laudable, but it can sometimes be a double-edged sword. While on the one hand, it acts as a shield, protecting us from external storms, on the other, it can cage us, silencing our innermost cries for help.

In the aftermath of life's tumultuous events, having grappled with the trauma of sexual assault and the heartbreak of divorce, I sensed an impending storm, potentially more terrifying than any I had faced before. Society's insistent whispers about resilience and bouncing back were a stark contrast to the fragmentation happening within me. It felt like I was a step away from a chasm, with a mental collapse waiting to claim me, as my mind wavered on the edge of a dark abyss.

It was during this time that depression sneaked into my life, silent and treacherous like a thief in the night, making its presence known in the most painfully real ways. I found myself engulfed in spontaneous bouts of crying, moments where the tears wouldn't stop, and all I wanted to do was lay still, wishing for the world to fade away, sometimes even contemplating the finality of death. The sheer effort to continue each day felt like an insurmountable climb.

Recognizing that these weren't just bad days, I sought professional help. The doctor's diagnosis confirmed my fears: I was clinically depressed. It wasn't just the sadness or a phase of grief; it was a real, consuming condition, validating the internal chaos that had been my unwelcome companion. Depression didn't knock before it entered; it just settled in like a fog that wouldn't lift, proving that mental health struggles like these are as real and tangible as any physical ailment. It marked the beginning of a new battle, one that required me to face this uninvited intruder head-on.

Amid this internal strife, the physical manifestations of this internal chaos were visceral. My nerves felt constantly under assault, as though a sharp pencil was being driven relentlessly onto the scalp of my head. Anxiety and panic attacks became frequent, uninvited guests, their grip so tight that even the simplest tasks became nearly impossible to manage.

I recall one particularly challenging night while driving home from work. I was on the phone with my sister-friend Betty when an intense anxiety attack overtook me. It was debilitating, and I was convinced a heart attack was imminent. Betty's voice was my only anchor as she stayed with me on the line, guiding me through the crippling panic until it subsided.

Night times, which should have been a refuge of rest, morphed into a theater of terror. I would spring out of bed, propelled by hallucinations of smoke, and find myself running aimlessly, trying to escape the imagined flames.

It became clear that I was on the brink of a nervous breakdown. My nerves were frayed, and in a desperate attempt to quell the unrest, I often turned to alcohol, seeking a reprieve from the relentless anxiety. However, the ultimate tipping point came when I recognized that I could no longer function in my professional capacity. I made the difficult decision to take a leave of absence from my job, understanding that my mental health had to be the priority. For six exhaustive weeks, I committed myself to outpatient therapy, a necessary step towards regaining control over the chaos that had hijacked my mind. It was during these sessions that I desperately tried to weave back together the unraveling threads of my mental well-being. During this period, medication became my lifeline. Pills to jolt me awake, pills to lull me into a restless slumber, and pills just to face the relentless march of hours. It was a crutch I hadn't anticipated needing, but in that period, they were indispensable.

And yet, despite the internal tempest, the world outside continued its incessant chant, "Stay strong. Push through. Soldier on." This external pressure, rather than being a source of encouragement, became another weight upon already burdened shoulders.

It was in this burden of pain that a profound realization dawned upon me. True strength wasn't about masking my pain or numbing my emotions. It was about acknowledging them, giving voice to them, and seeking the help I desperately needed. It was about understanding that sometimes, falling apart is the first step to rebuilding.

Our society often glorifies an unyielding facade of toughness, but it's in our brokenness, in our raw and vulnerable moments that we truly discover our depths. By embracing my fragility, seeking therapy, and sharing my struggles, I was, in essence, defying the societal norm. I was redefining strength on my terms.

In the face of overwhelming challenges, whether they be traumas from the past or present battles with mental health, "staying strong" isn't about concealing pain. It's about having the courage to face it head-on, to seek assistance when needed, and to understand that our strength is not diminished by our moments of vulnerability but rather amplified by them.

3 FROM TRIALS TO TRIUMPHS: TRANSFORMING CHALLENGES INTO CHANCES

~Challenges as Stepping Stones~

Have you ever tried assembling a puzzle? Those intricate pieces, each so distinct and seemingly random, often leave us bewildered at first. Yet, as we begin to connect them, piece by piece, a beautiful image emerges, making sense of the chaos. What seemed like an overwhelming challenge transformed into an artwork, a testament to our patience and perseverance.

Similarly, in the vast puzzle of life, we frequently face challenges that seem distinct and devastating. These challenges might manifest as unexpected setbacks, heartbreaks, or life-altering events. It's easy to view them as burdens, hurdles blocking our path to happiness and success. However, what if we began seeing these challenges not as obstructions but as crucial pieces of our life's puzzle?

In this chapter, we will explore the transformative power of perspective. Instead of viewing challenges as barriers, we'll learn to see them as stepping stones, each challenge elevating us, providing invaluable lessons, and molding our character. By shifting our mindset, we can transform adversities into advantages, turning life's trials into opportunities for growth and enlightenment.

Through a blend of personal tales and shared wisdom, this chapter aims to inspire resilience and determination. You'll discover that every challenge, no matter how daunting, carries with it the potential to shape, refine, and propel us forward. Let's dive into this journey of reimagining challenges, finding the silver linings, and turning life's toughest moments into our greatest assets.

~Reshaping Perspective: From Obstacles to Opportunities~

Life has a peculiar way of revealing a spectrum of experiences. Often, it is not the situations that alter, but our perspective towards them. As we journey through life, traversing its many twists and turns, our viewpoint plays a decisive role in shaping our reactions, actions, and, ultimately, our paths.

In my personal voyage, I've faced mountains, seemingly insurmountable. From the harrowing experiences of my past to the mental health battles that threatened to consume me, each challenge appeared as a blockade, an overwhelming barrier keeping me from my desired destination. But as I delved deeper into my own understanding and faith, an epiphany emerged. These obstacles, no matter how daunting, were not dead ends. They were detours, opportunities in disguise.

Take, for example, the biblical story of Joseph. Sold into slavery by his own brothers, wrongly accused, and thrown into prison, from an external viewpoint, his life seemed marred by a series of unfortunate events. Yet, through it all, Joseph's unwavering faith and ability to see God's hand in every circumstance turned his obstacles into opportunities. He went from being a prisoner to the second most powerful man in Egypt, saving nations from famine. It wasn't the absence of trials that defined Joseph's journey; it was his perspective during those trials.

In my struggles with mental health, societal pressures, and past traumas, I, too, had to undergo a transformative shift in perspective. Instead of viewing my moments of vulnerability and pain as definitive, I began to see them as transformative. My battles with anxiety and panic attacks, instead of being chains that bound me, became platforms on which I built my understanding, empathy, and renewed purpose. Every challenge became a lesson, every setback a setup for a comeback.

The therapy sessions, the sleepless nights, the pills that marked my days – they were not indicators of defeat. They became stepping stones, guiding me toward a future where I could leverage these experiences to inspire, uplift, and guide others. My obstacles were shaping me, molding me into a beacon of hope for others navigating similar turbulent waters.

In the mosaic of life, it's easy to get fixated on the broken pieces, on the sharp edges that seem to pierce our very souls. But with a change in perspective, those very pieces can be rearranged to form a beautiful, coherent whole. It's not about erasing or ignoring the challenges. It's about viewing them as integral parts of our unique journey, catalysts that propel us toward growth, understanding, and fulfillment.

As we traverse the various changes and phases of life, it's vital to bear in mind that it is our perspective, rather than our circumstances, that defines our path. By reshaping our viewpoint and transforming our mindset from perceiving obstacles to identifying opportunities, we don't merely endure; we thrive. As it says in Romans 12:2, "Do not conform to the patterns of this world but be transformed by the renewing of your mind." This scripture highlights the power of transforming our mindset to align with God's will and thrive in all circumstances.

~Personal Tales of Adversities Turned to Advantages~

If someone had told me years ago that one of the most heart-wrenching moments of my life would shape me into the resilient woman I am today, I would have met them with skepticism. Yet, the saga of my personal adversities ultimately became the chapters that defined my strength, ambition, and success. Unexpectedly becoming a single mother to three wonderful boys marked an unforeseen chapter in my life's book. Their young eyes, brimming with questions and concerns, served as my constant reminder that surrendering to my circumstances was not an option. Desperate to keep our home, I borrowed thousands from my parents, but the financial burdens became too much. With a heavy heart, I made the agonizing decision to let the house go into foreclosure and file for bankruptcy.

In the aftermath, we found solace in my parents' home. The walls of my childhood room, once adorned with dreams of youth, now cradled my small family as we navigated the aftermath of our upheaval. Watching my three boys adapt to this new normal, their resilience, confusion, hope, and heartbreak all intertwined, sparked a fire within me. I realized this moment of adversity could not be our defining moment; instead, it had to be our catalyst for transformation.

Drawing strength from a concept in Michelle Obama's profound memoir, "Becoming," which emphasizes that "Becoming requires equal parts patience and rigor," I embarked on a journey of transformation during my personal trials. This journey was not just for me but for the future and well-being of "my three sons." With renewed determination, I returned to school, burning the midnight oil, juggling coursework with motherhood, resolute to rewrite our narrative. The pride I felt upon obtaining my bachelor's degree was only eclipsed by the joy of achieving my master's. The same hands that once clutched divorce papers now held diplomas, tangible proof of my determination and resilience.

Simultaneously, my professional life thrived. I climbed the corporate ladder, each step a testament to my dedication, hard work, and the lessons learned from my adversities. Every advancement was not just for my career, it was for building a brighter future for my boys. I created a new, empowered life. My adversities, as distressing as they were, became my advantages. They instilled in me a vigor and determination I might never have discovered otherwise.

Who knew that the remnants of my past would be the fertile soil for my present? Who knew a shattered heart could give rise to such an unshakeable spirit? The story of my journey from despondency to triumph is a testament to the fact that our adversities, no matter how deterring, have the potential to propel us towards greatness. As I stand today, a pillar of strength for my sons, forged in the furnace of life's most challenging trials, I am grateful. For, as it is written in Romans 8:28 (NIV), "And we know that in all things God works for the good of those who love him, who have been called according to His purpose."

In the biblical story of Zelophehad's daughters, we see another powerful example of adversity turned to advantage. Zelophehad, a man from the Tribe of Manasseh, had five daughters and no sons. At that time, women were not entitled to inherit property, and the daughters of Zelophehad faced the prospect of losing their father's land. However, instead of accepting their fate, they petitioned Moses and the leaders of the Israelite community for the right to inherit their father's property. Their request was unprecedented, but it was granted, and it led to a change in the inheritance laws of ancient Israel, a significant victory not only for them but for all the daughters of Israel.

In the prism of my life, the most challenging experiences have crafted the most beautiful patterns. My journey, marked by the transformation of adversities into advantages, resonates instead with the wisdom of Michelle Obama from her memoir 'Becoming,' "Becoming isn't about arriving somewhere or achieving a certain aim. I see it instead as forward motion, a means of evolving, a way to reach continuously toward a better self. The journey doesn't end." And so, with a heart brimming with gratitude and a spirit fortified with strength, I move forward, ready to extend my love and newfound wisdom to others, turning the page to the next chapter of my journey.

~Techniques for Reframing Life's Setbacks~

Navigating life's journey, I now understand that our hurdles are not mere disruptions but potent lessons in disguise. Indeed, each challenge we face offers a profound opportunity for growth, self-discovery, and resilience. Much of this understanding and transformation stems from how we choose to perceive and address these challenges.

This became especially evident to me during a 21-day 'Keep It Moving Mindset Challenge' I participated in, led by Apostle Kimberly Jones. The challenge began with a reality check, an exercise that forced us to confront our current reality and be honest with ourselves about our situations. This initial step was crucial as it laid the groundwork for the subsequent stages of the challenge. Over the next 21 days, Apostle Jones pushed us to challenge our mindset in a very thought-provoking and introspective manner.

One of the key components that stood out to me in this challenge was the art of reframing. Reframing is the act of consciously shifting our perspective of a situation, allowing us to see it in a different light. It is an empowering practice that helps us view adversities as opportunities for growth rather than insurmountable problems. This concept became my sanctuary during the turbulent aftermath of my life's challenges. It was in this spirit of renewal and perspective shifts that I embraced several techniques to turn life's setbacks into pathways for personal evolution.

Here are five personal reframing techniques that can be applied in our day-to-day lives:

Embrace the New Normal

Accepting change is crucial. Instead of longing for the past or what could have been, focus on adapting and finding comfort in your new situation.

Growth Mindset

Adopt a growth mindset by viewing challenges as opportunities to learn and grow. This mindset will empower you to approach difficulties with a proactive and positive attitude.

Positive Self-Talk

Be mindful of the language you use when thinking or talking about yourself and your situation. Replace negative thoughts with positive affirmations to boost your confidence and resilience.

Visualize Success

Take time to visualize a positive outcome for your transition. Imagine yourself successfully navigating the challenges and emerging stronger on the other side.

Seek Support

Don't hesitate to lean on your support network or seek professional help if needed. Sharing your feelings and experiences with others can provide a fresh perspective and much-needed encouragement.

Embracing these practices has been transformative, helping me view my adversities as advantages and strengthening my resilience in the face of challenges. Apostle Kimberly Jones often emphasizes, "Your words have power, and you have the authority to change your narrative." Through the act of reframing and the application of these techniques, I have not only changed my narrative but also paved the way for a brighter, more empowered future.

4 FAITH IN THE MIDST OF FURY: GOD'S GUIDING HAND IN TURBULENT TIMES

~Finding God Amidst the Storm~

I recall a moment from years ago, standing by the window of my tiny apartment as rain pelted against the glass. The skies were dark, and thunder rumbled in the distance. It felt as if the world outside mirrored the turmoil inside my heart. But in the midst of that storm, as I looked at the droplets tracing paths down the window, I felt a strange comfort. It was as if each drop carried a message: that even amidst chaos, there's a pattern, a rhythm, a higher force at work.

Such moments of divine realization often come to us when we least expect them. When life throws us into the eye of the storm, when the ground beneath us seems to be shifting, it's easy to feel lost and detached from the spiritual. Yet, it's precisely in these moments of intense change or chaos that we can find God in the most profound ways.

In this chapter, we'll journey together into the depths of faith during tumultuous times. Drawing from personal experiences and moments of spiritual awakening, I'll share how I found solace, guidance, and strength by connecting with a higher power. Whether you're a devout believer or someone exploring spirituality, this chapter seeks to offer a beacon of hope, showcasing how God's presence can be felt even when clouds of doubt and despair loom large.

Join me as we navigate these spiritual waters, discovering how, even in our lowest moments, we can find signs, messages, and reassurances from the divine. Let's uncover the profound beauty of finding God amidst life's storms and learn how faith can be our anchor, grounding us through life's most turbulent transitions.

~ The Unyielding Embrace of Faith in Life's Whirlwinds ~

My deep affection for my church and its congregation was always the cornerstone of my existence. I relished the sense of belonging, the shared faith, and the fellowship with my church family. However, underneath that affection, there was a yearning for something greater, a desire for more of what God intended for me. The Bible tells us, "Now faith is confidence in what we hope for and assurance about what we do not see" (Hebrews 11:1). This scripture gained significant resonance when, in the early part of 2023, I found myself grappling with an unexpected inner turmoil while at the church. It felt akin to an out-of-body experience, where the joy and comfort that once came so naturally began to wane. I sensed that God understood my reluctance to make a proactive change, so it seemed He adjusted my circumstances, making my comfort zone increasingly uneasy and nudging me toward an unavoidable decision to depart. Exiting my home church after an astounding 48 years was an unexpected journey I had never envisioned. The walls, the wooden pews, the peace lilies gracing the background of the sermon podium, the delightful "Voices of Praise"- these were not mere material components or routine activities. They were integral elements ingrained deeply in my identity. While to those on the outside, it may have appeared merely a change of location, to me, it felt like relinquishing a piece of my soul.

The questions emerged relentlessly, a cacophony of confusion and self-doubt. Who was I without the familiar embrace of those beautiful clear glass windows and echoing hymn, "A charge to keep I have and a God to glorify?" Why was this profound change taking place now after nearly half a century of unwavering commitment? These were not just musings; they were agonizing cries from the very depths of my heart.

Few can truly fathom the agitated storm I found myself in. It wasn't just a mental or emotional tempest but one that manifested physically. Sleepless nights turned into exhausting days. My bed became both my refuge and my prison, with tear-streaked pillows bearing witness to my pain. I grieved deeply, not for bricks and stones, but for the spiritual family I had cultivated over decades. A family that prayed together, laughed and cried together, and, most importantly, grew in faith together.

Yet, amidst this churning sea of uncertainty, a steadfast anchor emerged: my unwavering faith. It wasn't an elixir that took away the pain, nor a wand that magically set things right. But it was an omnipresent force, gently nudging me, reminding me of God's grander scheme. A voice that softly whispered, even during those harrowing nights, that there was a purpose, a divine orchestration behind the transition I was experiencing.

To say that embracing my faith was the solution would be an oversimplification. Rather, it became my guiding compass, directing me through the dense fog of confusion. It was the hand I held when traversing this unfamiliar terrain, the warm embrace that sheltered me from the cold winds of doubt.

Faith assured me that while I might have left a place I dearly loved, I hadn't abandoned or been abandoned by God. He was there, just as He always had been, walking beside me, helping me chart a new spiritual journey. Through all the pain, the uncertainty, and the sleepless nights, faith remained my most loyal companion. It manifested profoundly the assurance found in Scripture: "Be strong and courageous. Do not be afraid or terrified because of them, for the Lord your God goes with you; he will never leave you nor forsake you." (Deuteronomy 31:6)

In retrospect, this trying phase wasn't just about loss or change; it was an evolution, a transition to a deeper and more intimate relationship with my faith. It reinforced the notion that buildings might define a congregation, but unwavering faith truly defines one's spiritual journey.

~God's Grand Design: Deciphering His Signs and Believing in His Ways~

Billy Graham beautifully captured the essence of faith when he remarked, "When we come to the end of ourselves, we come to the beginning of God." It's a profound reminder that, at the heart of uncertainty, the real journey begins, one of recognizing God's plans and entrusting ourselves to His process.

Life often has its way of unfolding in manners unexpected and sometimes undesired. In these intricacies of existence, we seek signs, looking for assurances that we're headed in the right direction or making the right decisions. But deciphering these signs can be challenging, especially when they are subtle and require a deep connection to our spiritual self.

From my earliest days, I can recall my mother's unwavering belief in Holy Spirit's guidance. She'd often say, "When in doubt, seek the Holy Spirit. It's the voice of God within you, guiding, reassuring, and directing." There was an absolute faith in her words, a deep-seated trust in the Spirit's wisdom. Growing up, she instilled in me the importance of this divine compass. Every time life pushed me to a corner, I would recall her words, seeking that inner voice, leaning on Holy Spirit's guidance.

The Holy Spirit, often considered our Advocate, illuminates our path with God's intentions. It's not about grand gestures or loud proclamations but the silent whispers, the inner nudges, and the peace it brings, even amidst turmoil. As Romans 8:26 beautifully articulates, "In the same way, the Spirit helps us in our weakness. We do not know what we ought to pray for, but the Spirit himself intercedes for us through wordless groans." In times of doubt and despair, I've often felt these wordless groans, an unspoken connection that fills the void, reminding me of God's unwavering presence.

Believing in God's divine plan means trusting a design greater than our understanding. It's about seeing beyond the immediate and recognizing the long-term blessings that God has in store. A favored scripture of mine that underlines this faith is Proverbs 16:9, "A man's heart plans his way, but the Lord directs his steps." Our journey might be filled with plans, detours, and unexpected stops, but it's the Lord who ensures each step aligns with His grand design.

Embracing God's divine plan, recognizing His signs, and yielding to the guidance of Holy Spirit doesn't guarantee a smooth path, but it does promise a journey filled with purpose, love, and divine support. As we navigate life's transitions and seek clarity amidst chaos, let us remember my mother's wisdom, lean into the embrace of Holy Spirit, and trust that every step, every moment, is a beautiful, purposeful addition to God's magnificent design for our lives. Thanks, Mom.

~Divine Interventions: From Empty Jars to Scarlet Threads~

Life often presents us with unexpected turns, moments when our well-laid plans seem to crumble, leaving us in a state of confusion and despair. Yet, within these moments of seeming interruption, if we choose to see with eyes of faith, we may discern the fingerprints of divine intervention, gently guiding us toward our destined purpose. The scriptures brim with stories of individuals who, in the face of obstacles, found that life's interruptions didn't thwart their purpose, but instead, enhanced it.

Take, for example, the narrative of Elisha and the widow as recorded in 2 Kings 4:1-7. The widow, with debts piling up and facing the prospect of her sons being taken away as slaves, was on the brink of utter despair. She had nothing left but a small jar of oil. Enter the prophet Elisha, who instructed her to gather as many empty jars as she could and pour out her meager supply of oil into them. Miraculously, the oil didn't run out until she had filled every vessel. From the brink of destitution, the widow was propelled into a place of provision, not just for the immediate crisis, but for her future. The interruption of debt and imminent loss was transformed into an opportunity for divine provision and miraculous multiplication.

In the same spirit of unexpected divine intervention, we find the story of Rahab in the book of Joshua 2:1-21. Rahab, a prostitute in the city of Jericho, would be perceived by many as living a life interrupted by poor choices and societal disdain. Yet, when Israelite spies entered her city, she recognized the hand of God upon their nation and chose to assist them. By hiding the spies and later letting them escape, Rahab secured a promise of safety for herself and her family. What's more striking is that Rahab's story didn't end with the fall of Jericho. She was woven into the very lineage of Jesus Christ, a testament to how one's past or profession doesn't define one's divine purpose.

Both these narratives, though set in vastly different contexts, underscore a profound truth: life's interruptions, be it through external circumstances or personal choices, don't necessarily cancel out our purpose. In fact, they might be the very platforms upon which our true purpose is unveiled.

In my journey, I've encountered numerous interruptions, moments when the road ahead seemed obscured. Yet, with time and perspective, I've come to recognize that these moments, rather than diverging me from my path, were guiding me toward a deeper understanding of my purpose. Like the widow, there have been times of lack where resources seemed scant. Yet, in those very moments, I've witnessed provisions, both tangible and intangible, flow into my life in unexpected abundance. And akin to Rahab, there were instances where past mistakes loomed large, casting shadows on the present. But even in those shadows, glimmers of divine purpose broke through, reminding me that my story was still being written, and every chapter, every interruption, was part of a grander narrative.

In the end, the stories of Elisha and the widow, Rahab, and countless others from the annals of faith teach us a valuable lesson: interruptions are not dead ends but detours that lead us to divine encounters and deeper revelations of our purpose.

5 STEADFAST AMIDST THE SHIFTING SANDS: BUILDING RESILIENCE & FORTITUDE

~The Pillars of Resilience and Fortitude~

As I sat by the tranquil waters of a serene lake one cool evening, I found myself lost in thought, reflecting on the ripples that spread outward with every stone I tossed in. These ripples, though momentarily disruptive, didn't unsettle the lake's core. The water returned to its calm state, resilient against the brief disturbances. In that moment, it struck me: aren't we, too, much like that lake, facing countless ripples in the journey of life?

Each of us has faced moments when life's stones—be they challenges, heartbreaks, or setbacks—have disrupted our tranquility. And while these moments may have left us momentarily shaken, there exists within each of us a reservoir of resilience and fortitude, allowing us to find our calm amidst the chaos.

In this introspective chapter, we will dive deep into the very essence of these two pillars—resilience and fortitude. Drawing from moments of self-reflection, experiences from my own life, and the wisdom of countless others who've walked similar paths, we'll explore how these inner strengths can be nurtured, cultivated, and harnessed.

Together, we will seek to understand the true meaning of resilience—not just as the ability to bounce back but to grow through adversity. We'll also reflect on the nature of fortitude, that quiet inner strength that enables us to hold our ground even when the winds of change threaten to topple us.

Join me in this meditative exploration as we unearth the depths of our resilience and fortitude. As we journey together, I hope this chapter offers you a mirror, allowing you to see and recognize the incredible strength that has always resided within you, waiting to guide you through life's ripples and waves.

~ Cultivating Inner Strength and Endurance ~

In a world filled with uncertainties, the only surefire way to triumph over life's many adversities is by cultivating inner strength and endurance. Often, we admire individuals who seem to have it all figured out, completely overlooking the resilience and fortitude that undergird their accomplishments.

However, as we peel back the layers of their journeys, we discover that these attributes are not just essential but are, in fact, the bedrock upon which their success is built.

The biblical story of Hannah is a striking example of resilience and fortitude. Hannah, one of two wives of a man named Elkanah, was unable to have children. In a society where a woman's value was often measured by her ability to bear offspring, this was a crushing blow. Year after year, she faced humiliation and taunts from Peninnah, Elkanah's other wife, who had children of her own. The pain of her barrenness was compounded by the constant reminder of her perceived inadequacy. Nevertheless, Hannah refused to succumb to despair.

Hannah's journey was marked by relentless prayer and an unwavering faith in God. Year after year, she poured out her heart to the Lord, laying bare her deepest desires and pain. Despite the ridicule, the disappointment, and the seemingly insurmountable odds, Hannah remained steadfast. Her endurance was not merely a passive waiting but an active and fervent seeking of God's favor. Hannah's story culminates in a powerful moment when she makes a vow to the Lord, promising that if He gives her a son, she will dedicate him to the Lord's service. God honors her faith and grants her request, resulting in the birth of Samuel, who would go on to be one of Israel's greatest prophets.

Hannah's story is not just about the power of prayer, but it is a testament to the strength that can be found in resilience and fortitude. She teaches us that enduring hardship is not merely weathering the storm but actively seeking growth and transformation amidst the challenges. Hannah did not allow her circumstances to define her; instead, she found strength in her faith and devotion to God.

As we navigate our own journeys, we must cultivate a similar sense of resilience and fortitude. Life will undoubtedly throw curveballs our way, and there will be moments when it feels as though all hope is lost. However, by embracing the lessons learned from Hannah's journey, we can develop an inner strength that enables us to persevere and, ultimately, triumph over adversity.

Fostering inner fortitude and persistence is more than a singular achievement; it's a perpetual journey that necessitates purposeful engagement. This concept is compellingly personified through the experiences of African American social justice activist Rosa Parks. Her life wasn't about a single act of defiance on a Montgomery bus but a lifelong commitment to growth and equality in the face of systemic adversity.

Rosa Parks' circumstances were steeped in the challenges posed by racial segregation. Yet, she didn't perceive these challenges as unconquerable giants. Instead, she saw them as opportunities for societal improvement and personal empowerment. Rather than concentrating on the freedoms and rights she was denied, she positioned her mindset on the potential positive changes her actions and courage could help realize.

She embraced a perspective that underscored potential gains over present losses — a mindset that eventually played a significant role in the civil rights movement. Her decision to remain seated was not about what was taken from her in that moment, but what could be gained for countless others in the future: the right to equality and freedom from oppression.

Most critically, Rosa Parks' journey involved an unwavering commitment to self-improvement and communal advancement, persisting even when faced with intimidation, threats, and discrimination. Her story is a testament to the continuous process of cultivating resilience. It's about the relentless pursuit of growth opportunities, both personally and for the greater good, despite the towering barriers of adversity. Her resolve and the subsequent transformative actions didn't just symbolize endurance; they epitomized the power of sustained, forward-thinking effort and resilience in the continual quest for a just and equitable society.

As we journey through life, let us strive to emulate Rosa's and Hannah's resilience and fortitude. Let us commit to cultivating an inner strength that enables us to face challenges head-on and emerge stronger on the other side. And, in doing so, let us remember that our true power lies not in our ability to avoid adversity but in our capacity to overcome it.

~Harness Resilience During Transitions Hagar's Way~

Years ago, I conceptualized an event that would not only bear witness to my personal journey but also serve as a beacon of hope for many women navigating the tempestuous waters of life. The "Find Your Fortitude: Women's Conference" was more than just a gathering; it was a testament to the incredible strength and resilience that lies dormant within each of us, waiting for the right moment to awaken.

Behind this conference was a narrative personal to me. Though I was its creator, the inspiration came from my reflection of being a single parent. At the time, the meager salary from my entry-level position at a reputable company was barely enough to support myself, let alone my three "hungry" young boys.

To add to the strain, the court granted me a mere $150 per month for child support for all three of them. During this time, a phrase became a constant refrain in my mind, echoing my sentiments: "I hate it here."

In the deafening noise of my struggles, a biblical story spoke to me–the story of Hagar. An Egyptian maidservant, Hagar faced circumstances that were beyond her control. After bearing Abraham's child, she was mistreated and finally driven into the desert. Alone, scared, and with a child to care for, Hagar must have felt the weight of the world upon her. Yet, even in her anguish, she encountered God. He not only acknowledged her pain, but He also promised her a lineage as vast as the stars. Hagar's story resonated with my journey. Her despair, resilience, and unyielding faith in the Almighty mirrored my own experiences.

Single parenting is a journey fraught with challenges. And single parenting three boys? It demands not just strength, but a fortitude carved from the very bedrock of our being. I had plans, dreams of a future where my children and I would rise above our current circumstances. But these weren't mere daydreams; they demanded action. During this phase, I often felt God guiding me, offering strategies and a path to harness my inner resilience: like how He guided Hagar through her desert.

Through my faith, I realized that my struggles were not a sign of abandonment but a testament to God's faith in my strength, much like Hagar's desert was not her end but a transition to a destiny grander than she could imagine. The weight of the world, though heavy, was not unbearable; it was a challenge, pushing me to discover the depths of my strength and resilience.

My "Find Your Fortitude: Women's Conference" was a culmination of these revelations. It was an ode to all the Hagars of the world, every woman who has faced the harshest deserts of life and emerged stronger, more resilient. As women shared their stories, the atmosphere was charged with an energy of hope and strength.

Today, as I reflect on my journey and that of countless other women, I am reminded of a simple truth: life's deserts are not barren wastelands but grounds for transformation. With faith as our compass and resilience as our guide, we can and will chart a path to our promised destiny.

~Spiritual Techniques for Grounding Oneself During Times of Distraction~

In my life, when the tides of change sought to pull me under, it was my faith that anchored me. The challenges I faced weren't merely external; they were inner storms, wrestling matches of the soul. But amidst the swirling chaos, a series of spiritual practices became my lifelines, guiding me back to a space of tranquility and a deeper connection with my Lord and Savior, Jesus Christ.

Prayer

More than a ritual, prayer was my intimate dialogue with the Almighty. When the weight of the world bore down on me, I found solace in the quiet conversations, whispering my fears and hopes into God's receptive ears. Through prayer, I felt heard and understood. The words of Philippians 4:6-7 became a mantra: "Do not be anxious about anything, but in every situation, by prayer and petition, with thanksgiving, present your requests to God. And the peace of God, which transcends all understanding, will guard your hearts and minds in Christ Jesus."

Meditation

Many perceive meditation as a secular practice, but I found it deeply spiritual. By silencing my thoughts, I could better hear the gentle whispers of God. Meditation allowed me to dwell in His presence, absorbing His love, grace, and guidance.

The Word of God

The Bible isn't just a book to me; it is a treasure trove of wisdom, stories, and lessons. Diving deep into its pages, I felt the narratives come alive, speaking directly to my situation. Scriptures like Psalm 46:10, "Be still, and know that I am God," became sources of strength, reassuring me of God's omnipresence during my trials.

Spending Time with God

Beyond structured rituals, I reserved moments in my day akin to spending time with a dear friend just to be with God. It could be a walk in the park, reflecting on His wonders, or simply sitting in silence, basking in His love. This unhurried, unstructured time created a profound bond, making me more attuned to His voice in my daily life.

Relying on God for Strength

Every setback, every tear shed, became an opportunity to lean into God's enduring strength. Isaiah 41:10 became a beacon, "So do not fear, for I am with you; do not be dismayed, for I am your God. I will strengthen you and help you; I will uphold you with my righteous right hand."

Fasting

Fasting, for me, was more than abstaining from food; it was a deep, spiritual cleansing. It was a way to declutter, to shift my focus entirely onto God. It made my prayers more fervent and my connection more profound. Matthew 6:17-18 reminded me, "But when you fast, put oil on your head and wash your face, so that it will not be obvious to others that you are fasting, but only to your Father, who is unseen; and your Father, who sees what is done in secret, will reward you."

Reflecting on my past, I recognize now that these spiritual practices provided more than just comfort in times of turmoil; they fundamentally altered how I view life's hurdles. I learned to perceive difficulties not as overwhelming barriers but as instigators of spiritual evolution. With each tempest, my faith became more profound, my connection with the Divine more robust, and I reemerged each time more polished and resilient than before. Though the world around me perpetually changes, having God with me ensures my spirit stands steadfast.

6 RIDING LIFE'S EMOTIONAL WAVES: ACHIEVING BALANCE IN THE CHAOS

~Navigating Emotional Upheavals~

As a child, one of my most cherished memories was the trips my father would take me on to Six Flags Over Georgia. The Mind Bender was my absolute favorite roller coaster. Each time I climbed onto that ride; I would feel a surge of adrenaline. The anticipation during the climb, the rush of the wind on my face during the descent, and the unpredictability of the twists and turns would fill me with both exhilaration and a sense of trepidation. It was a thrilling experience, yet it also drained me emotionally, leaving me feeling simultaneously revitalized and depleted. Isn't it intriguing how this roller coaster journey mirrors life itself, with its alternating periods of emotional peaks and valleys?

Emotions, much like that roller coaster, have the power to sweep us off our feet, taking us on journeys of joy, sorrow, elation, and despair. And while these emotional journeys are integral to the human experience, navigating the tumultuous waves of feelings is seldom straightforward.

In this chapter, we will explore the complex realm of emotions with the goal of improving our ability to comprehend, control, and direct our emotional reactions during periods of change. By referencing personal stories and expert opinions, we will examine approaches to keep our emotions in check, even amidst the surrounding chaos.

Together, we'll embark on a journey to uncover the roots of our most profound emotions, learning to accept them as natural, valid, and deeply human. By understanding the triggers and patterns of our emotional responses, we can better prepare ourselves to face life's transitions with grace and equanimity.

As you turn these pages, consider them a guide to your inner emotional landscape—a map to help you chart a course through the unpredictable seas of feelings. Let's navigate these waters together, seeking clarity, balance, and a deeper connection to our emotional selves.

~Understanding and Accepting Our Emotional Spectrum~

The heart is an extraordinary vessel. It is where we store our joys and sorrows, our triumphs and regrets. Just as the sky presents a medley of hues from the deepest blues to the radiant oranges, our emotional landscape, too, paints a vivid spectrum, spanning the depths of despair to the peaks of elation.

As a child, I was taught there were "good" and "bad" emotions. Joy, enthusiasm, and gratitude were welcomed, while anger, sadness, and jealousy were frowned upon and dismissed as mere inconveniences that were best pushed away. But life, in its infinite wisdom, taught me that this compartmentalization was far too simplistic.

One evening, as I sat in my office, a flood of memories from a past event came rushing back. The sharp sting of betrayal, the weight of disappointment, the cold embrace of loneliness. These feelings had been buried deep, away from the conscious realm. But that evening, they demanded recognition. Instead of pushing them away as I usually did, I allowed myself to truly feel. I let the tears flow, the heartache throb, and the anger surge.

In that raw, vulnerable state, I turned to my faith. I whispered a prayer, not for the pain to vanish, but for the strength to understand it. And in that silent conversation, a realization dawned upon me: My emotions, whether deemed 'positive' or 'negative,' were all integral facets of my human experience.

They weren't chains that held me back but were, in fact, teachers in their own right.

Anger taught me about boundaries, pointing out where mine had been crossed. Sadness was a testament to my ability to love and form deep connections. Jealousy highlighted areas of my own insecurities and where I needed to focus my personal growth.

Embracing my emotional spectrum wasn't about succumbing to chaos. It was about achieving genuine clarity. When I permitted myself to feel without judgment, I began to understand myself better. Psalm 139:14 says, "I praise you, for I am fearfully and wonderfully made." Indeed, our emotional depth and complexity are not mistakes but divine designs.

The journey toward understanding and embracing my emotions was anything but straightforward. It featured moments of refusal to acknowledge my feelings and times of confusion. However, through steadfastness, I slowly mastered the art of navigating my emotional realms with grace. What once seemed like overwhelming torrents evolved into waves I learned to maneuver. This shift in my approach and reaction to my emotions was significantly shaped by a principle imparted by Apostle Kimberly Jones, which is to "Feel the feeling, choose the behavior." This powerful adage reminded me to fully recognize and immerse myself in my emotions, while simultaneously being mindful and deliberate in my responses to them.

In our quest for eternal happiness, we often forget that growth stems from embracing all facets of our emotions. The valleys make the peaks more profound. The rainy days make the sunny ones shine brighter. And as I stood there, acknowledging, feeling, and understanding, I wasn't just reconnecting with myself; I was deepening my bond with the Creator who had, in His infinite wisdom, crafted this beautiful, intricate emotional palette within me.

~Practical Exercises for Emotional Balance and Well-being~

If we consider our emotions as the colors used to paint our life's journey, mastering our emotional state is like producing a compelling and unforgettable film. Over time, I've understood that achieving emotional balance is not about quieting certain emotions over others. Instead, it involves giving each emotion its rightful role, allowing for a symphony of feelings that create a cohesive whole. Similar to a director shaping a film, I had to learn to navigate, balance, and deploy my emotions with purpose and discernment.

This principle is powerfully embodied in the film "Harriet," which chronicles the extraordinary life of Harriet Tubman, an iconic African American freedom fighter. The movie captures the complex range of emotions that Harriet experiences and harnesses in her courageous journey from slavery to becoming a conductor on the Underground Railroad and, eventually, a legendary abolitionist. Amidst fear, uncertainty, and danger, Harriet feels an array of emotions, from despair to hope, rage to love, each serving a purpose in her mission.

Throughout "Harriet," emotional wellness is not depicted as merely having positive feelings. Instead, Harriet's strength comes from her ability to acknowledge, accept, and utilize each emotion in her challenging path. For instance, her fear is not suppressed but transformed into caution and vigilance during her perilous missions to lead slaves to freedom. Her anger at the injustice of slavery fuels her passion and determination to fight for freedom.

The movie demonstrates that mastering our emotions means allowing each one to play its part in our life narratives, contributing to our overall resilience and purpose. Harriet's journey is a testament to the fact that true emotional balance requires each feeling to be felt and understood, contributing to the richness of our human experience. In her life's movie, every emotion was a critical scene, driving her forward and shaping her destiny, teaching viewers that our emotions can be powerful instruments of change when embraced and guided wisely.

Reflecting on this, my personal journey mirrors Harriet's in a way. The initial attempts to navigate the complex terrain of my emotions were anything but clean and orderly. There were moments of being completely swamped, with the various shades of my feelings intermingling and leaving behind a confused array of colors. Yet, much like Harriet, I learned that perseverance was key. With continued effort and the integration of certain strategies, what once was a tumultuous whirl of colors started to manifest as a clear, understandable image.

Journaling

Putting pen to paper has been one of the most transformative practices I've adopted. The act of documenting my feelings allowed me to step back and observe them from a distance. Over time, patterns emerged, and I could proactively address recurring emotional triggers, understanding their roots and navigating them with greater ease.

Mindful Breathing

The beauty of this exercise is its simplicity. Whenever I felt a surge of intense emotion, I'd pause, close my eyes, and take five deep breaths. This practice anchored me, allowing the storm of feelings to pass, granting clarity and calmness in its wake.

Emotion Mapping

Inspired by a therapy session, I began to physically map out my emotions. On a piece of paper, I'd draw circles representing different feelings, their size corresponding to their intensity. This visual representation was a revelation. It provided a snapshot of my emotional landscape at any given time, making intangible feelings tangible and manageable.

Setting Intentions

Every morning, before the day's hustle took over, I'd set an emotional intention. Whether it was patience, joy, gratitude, or understanding, this act of choosing my dominant feeling for the day gave me a sense of control and purpose.

Gratitude Rituals

On particularly challenging days, I'd turn to my gratitude jar. Filled with small notes of daily blessings and joys, this jar was a reminder of the good that coexisted alongside the challenges. Reading a few notes would instantly uplift my spirits, offering perspective and balance.

Nature Walks

There's something inherently therapeutic about nature. The rhythmic chirping of birds, the rustle of leaves, and the vastness of the skies all served as gentle reminders of the world's beauty and my small yet significant place within it. Regular walks in nature became my sanctuary: a space where emotions could flow freely, finding their natural equilibrium.

As days turned into weeks and weeks into months, these practices slowly but surely started to yield results. My emotional landscape, once tumultuous and unpredictable, began to resemble a serene, balanced painting filled with depth, variety, and harmony.

The pursuit of emotional well-being is a continuous process. Like an artist forever perfecting his craft, I, too, am learning, evolving, and refining my techniques. But with these tools in hand, I'm confident of my ability to manage the complex feelings that make up the human experience, crafting a life filled with balance, understanding, and profound beauty.

~The Imperative of Emotional Balance and Well-being During Transitions~

From those moments of meditation and contemplation, when I anchored myself through scripture and the whisper of prayer, I emerged with more than just spiritual grounding. I had a toolkit–practical exercises for emotional balance and well-being. Yet, with every tool at my disposal, I was soon to realize that knowledge alone wasn't enough. Implementing these tools during real-life transitions would become my most significant challenge and lesson.

Bishop T.D. Jakes once insightfully remarked, "If you can't figure out your purpose, figure out your passion. For your passion will lead you right into your purpose." As I found myself at the crossroads of yet another life transition, these words echoed in my heart. The tools I had gathered weren't just strategies; they were a means to an end, and avenue to channel my passion and subsequently discover and reaffirm my purpose.

The unpredictability of life changes brought with it a cascade of emotions. At times, joy and hope would burgeon, painting my world in bright hues. Yet, at other moments, the canvas of my heart was streaked with the somber shades of anxiety and fear. It was in these oscillations that the importance of emotional balance came to the fore.

The shifting sands of transition can unsettle the sturdiest of souls. But equipped with my newfound tools and an understanding of their importance, I began the delicate dance of engaging with my emotions. By asking myself the reasons behind each feeling, I could discern their messages and use them as guiding beacons.

But let's be candid; the journey wasn't always smooth sailing. There were phases of tumult, days when the weight of my emotions threatened to pull me under. Yet, with the dual power of spiritual anchoring and my practical toolkit, I charted a course through the stormy seas of transition.

In essence, while spiritual grounding provides the compass, emotional balance ensures the resilience to navigate life's transitions. And as Bishop T.D. Jakes so aptly highlighted in aligning our passions with purpose, particularly amidst life's challenges, we not only survive but thrive, finding clarity amidst the chaos.

~ The Therapeutic Power of Sharing and Connection During Transitions~

I often find myself reminiscing in the quiet moments, with the soft glow of my reading lamp casting long shadows over the room, flicking through the pages of old journals. These pages, worn from the grip of contemplative fingers, are a testament to the many transitions life has thrust upon me. From moments of triumphant highs to harrowing lows, it's all chronicled here. But as I trace through the words, an evolution is evident — a journey from solitude to sharing, from containment to connection.

In the earlier chapters of my life, when I grappled with mental health issues, I found solace in outpatient therapy, a sanctuary where I discovered a community not bound by shared hobbies or interests but by shared experiences. It was a space where vulnerability wasn't merely accepted; it was cherished and nurtured. During my initial visits, I found myself listening more than speaking, drawing courage and strength from the brave souls around me who bared their hearts and shared their narratives. Each person's journey was a testament to resilience, a beacon of hope in the sometimes-melancholic symphony of life.

The time finally came when it was my turn to speak. The room, pregnant with anticipation, seemed to hang on to every word as I unraveled my story. The freedom I found in releasing my truth, my testimony, was liberating and therapeutic. With each spoken word, I felt lighter, as if years of emotional baggage were being left behind. What was astounding was the ripples my story created. Eyes that once mirrored pain now gleamed with hope, and silent nods of understanding echoed the sentiment: "You're not alone."

This transformative power of vulnerability brings to mind another biblical example, Deborah. Found in the Book of Judges, Deborah was a woman of exceptional faith and leadership. As a prophetess and the lone female judge during a challenging period in Israel's history, she stepped into her role with unwavering trust, not in her own abilities, but in the divine guidance of God.

Much like Deborah, I've come to understand the profound impact of sharing one's personal journey for a purpose greater than oneself. By opening up about my own trials and victories, I've not only found personal healing, but I have also offered solace, strength, and a sense of belonging to others. As I continued to share, I discovered that God was opening doors for me to connect with a broader audience. My testimony transformed into a source of hope for many.

Think of life as a grand symphony, where each instrument, no matter how unique, contributes to the harmonious composition. When we share our life's music with the world, we realize that our individual stories are integral notes in this magnificent opus, where each of us has a role to play and a message to convey.

Our narratives and testimonies become more than personal records; they are catalysts for change. Just as Deborah's story inspires us with her unwavering faith and courage, our stories remind us and those we share them with that even in the darkest moments, a new day awaits. Through the power of vulnerability and connection, we not only heal and rejuvenate ourselves but also touch the lives of countless others, encouraging them to embrace their inner strength and share it with the world.

7 PHOENIX RISING: CHARTING A COURSE FROM DESOLATION TO HOPE

~Rebuilding After Setbacks~

There's an ancient parable about a phoenix, a mythical bird that rises anew from its own ashes. After a lifetime of radiant flight, the phoenix is consumed by flames, reduced to mere ashes. Yet, from those very ashes, it finds the strength to be reborn, soaring with renewed vigor and beauty. The story of the phoenix is not just a tale of rebirth but a testament to the unparalleled strength found in moments of profound transformation.

I've encountered moments in my life when everything appeared to turn to dust, dreams crumbled, hopes faded, and the future cast in shadow. It's during these somber times, when all seems lost, that the true process of reconstruction commences. This journey is neither swift nor without its share of pain, but within this forge of transformation, we unearth our profound wellsprings of strength and purpose.

In this chapter, we'll journey together through the painstaking yet empowering process of rebuilding after life's most crushing setbacks. Through raw, personal stories and hard-earned insights, we'll explore the steps to piece together a life broken by adversity, drawing lessons from personal experiences and the timeless wisdom of those who've walked similar paths.

We will delve deep into the strategies for forging a renewed sense of purpose, rekindling hope, and laying the foundation for a brighter, more resilient future. This chapter is a testament to the indomitable human spirit and the innate ability each one of us possesses to rise, rebuild, and rediscover our path after life's fiercest storms.

Join me in this authentic exploration as we learn not just to reconstruct what was lost but to fashion something even more beautiful from the remnants of our past. Remember, like the phoenix, it's never too late to rise from the ashes, redefine our destiny, and soar to new heights.

~Finding Hope and Purpose in the Aftermath of Despair~

In the shadows of despair, where hope seems lost, and the weight of life's trials feels overwhelming, lies the potential for profound spiritual growth and understanding. This chapter explores such a journey through the life of Job, a man whose story embodies enduring faith amidst life's harshest storms.

Job's story, as chronicled in the Book of Job, begins with a life marked by prosperity and piety. "There was a man in the land of Uz, whose name was Job; and that man was blameless and upright, and one who feared God and shunned evil" (Job 1:1). Yet, in an instant, this life of tranquility was shattered, as Job faced unimaginable losses–his livestock, his servants, and tragically, his children (Job 1:13-19).

I, like many, have found myself in similar valleys of despair, where the pain and confusion feel all-consuming. Job's reaction resonates deeply with us when he says, "The Lord gave, and the Lord has taken away; Blessed be the name of the Lord" (Job 1:21). His ability to acknowledge his pain yet still praise God is a profound lesson in faith.

As Job's trials continued, with painful sores afflicting his body (Job 2:7), his struggle to understand the 'why' behind his suffering became more pronounced. This quest for answers is something we all face in our darkest hours. Job's heartfelt lament, "Why did I not die at birth?" (Job 3:11), echoes the depth of despair that can cloud our hearts.

Job's friends, in their attempts to offer comfort, initially sat with him in silent support (Job 2:13). However, as time passed, their words turned to criticism and judgment, reflecting a common human error of misinterpreting suffering as punishment. In our own lives, the words, and actions of those around us can either be a source of comfort or a further test of our faith.

Despite the immense suffering and the well-intentioned but misguided counsel of his friends, Job's faith remained unshaken. He declared, "Though He slay me, yet will I trust Him" (Job 13:15). It's in this unwavering trust in God's plan, even when it's beyond our understanding, that we find true strength.

The pivotal moment in Job's story comes with God's response, not with explanations or justifications, but with questions that remind us of our limited understanding of the divine plan. "Where were you when I laid the foundations of the earth?" (Job 38:4). In my own journey, I've found solace in recognizing that some questions may remain unanswered, and that's where faith fills the gap.

Job's story concludes not just with the restoration of his fortunes but with a deeper, more intimate understanding and relationship with God. "My ears had heard of you but now my eyes have seen you" (Job 42:5). This transformation is not just about the restoration of material wealth or health but signifies a profound spiritual awakening.

In our lives, like Job's, despair can be a catalyst for growth and deepening faith. The path may be fraught with confusion and pain, yet it is also where we learn to truly trust God's plan. In the aftermath of despair, we don't just find hope and purpose; we discover a deeper connection with the Divine, an understanding that our journey, with all its ups and downs, is under His watchful eye.

The life of Job teaches us that amidst the greatest trials, our faith can guide us towards a deeper understanding and a renewed relationship with God. It reminds us that even when all seems lost, hope and purpose can be found in the unwavering belief that God is with us through every transition of life.

~Creating a Roadmap for Recovery and Rebirth~

In the wake of despair, after recognizing the strength of sharing and connection, a revelation surfaced. Once we have found hope and purpose in our tribulations, what follows? How do we shift from merely enduring to truly flourishing? To me, the road ahead involved not only progressing but doing so with deliberate intent and a sense of direction. This required crafting a blueprint for recovery and renewal.

Reflecting on my darkest hours, it seemed as though I was journeying through dense, unyielding mist. The way forward was hidden and fraught with uncertainty. However, as the fog of despair started to lift with the advent of newfound hope, the contours of a path began to take shape. This path was not solely about distancing myself from pain but steering towards a life filled with purpose and passion.

A crucial milestone in this blueprint was self-reflection. Engaging deeply in introspection, I discerned patterns and triggers, comprehending the 'whys' of past choices and the 'hows' of future ones. Journaling became my guiding compass, assisting in keeping tabs on where I had ventured and where I aimed to journey.

Subsequently came the crucial bridge of forgiveness. It was at this juncture I realized harboring resentment was akin to grasping a burning ember, hoping it would singe someone else. In truth, it was searing me from the inside. By letting go of these emotions, not only towards others, but also towards myself, I lightened my burdens for the road ahead.

Another pivotal turn was the lane of establishing boundaries. Acknowledging that prioritizing my well-being was permissible, I mastered the art of declining without guilt. These boundaries were not barriers but safeguarding measures, preserving the sanctity of my emotional and mental space.

The blueprint was not void of hurdles. There were deviations and stumbling blocks, but the focus remained steadfast on the destination. Along the way, mentors and guides materialized, often in unanticipated forms: a serendipitous book, a stranger's narrative, or even a soul-stirring melody. Each bestowed wisdom and enriched the blueprint.

Fundamentally, devising this blueprint transcended mere strategizing; it symbolized a rebirth. It entailed gathering the remnants of despair and piecing them together into a tapestry of hope, resilience, and purpose. As I embarked on this voyage, each step and each landmark broadened the horizon of possibilities, heralding a future aglow with promise and potential.

My passion for travel and having journeyed to various countries across the globe had instilled in me a "compass ready" mentality, a readiness to face the unknown with a plan, yet also with an openness to the unexpected. This mindset, coupled with the lessons from my past, equipped me to not just survive the journey but to thrive along the way.

~Gathering Resources and Seeking Support for a Fresh Start~

Following the charted path toward recovery and renewal, I quickly understood that navigating this journey would demand more than just self-driven determination. The subsequent phase involved arming myself with the essential tools and assembling a support network fundamental to my new beginning.

The baggage from my past, laden with memories of despair and challenges, was hefty. Simply laying it down was insufficient; I needed to unpack it, sift through its contents, and determine what to retain and what to relinquish. This unpacking prompted me to seek professional coaching. My coach, Coach BJ (yes, coaches have coaches), became a steadfast ally, helping me navigate the complex maze of my emotions and assisting in distinguishing what fueled my growth from what impeded it.

While coaching facilitated introspection, my soul craved connection. I participated in support groups and community gatherings, where narratives of struggles and victories resonated. The acknowledgment that I was not isolated, that many were confronting battles akin to mine, was immensely comforting. Each person's story contributed to my wellspring of strength. Their triumphs fueled my motivation, and their obstacles became lessons in resilience.

Remarkably, the most unanticipated support originated from my own network. Friends and family, whom I had inadvertently distanced myself from during my turbulent times, gradually returned. Their belief in my journey, even when I faltered, became the wind that lifted me. They reminded me of my identity before the storm and the person I could become after it.

To bolster this emotional and social support, I pursued informational resources. My shelves brimmed with books on personal development, spiritual healing, and even financial planning. Each page turned symbolized a stride towards autonomy and self-sufficiency.

Additionally, I sought spiritual guidance from Apostle Kimberly Jones and Pastor Natasha Rockmore, two women of God whose wisdom and encouragement that have been invaluable in my journey.

Moreover, I found inspiration in the story of Queen Esther from the Bible. Her courage, wisdom, and faith in the face of daunting challenges inspired me to approach my own obstacles with similar strength and determination.

Lastly, I embraced faith. In tranquil moments, when doubt would infiltrate, I would find a secluded spot, close my eyes, and seek comfort in prayer. This direct connection to the divine served as my anchor, stabilizing me when the world seemed tumultuous.

As I stood on the threshold of my new beginning, I was not solitary. I was enveloped by a plethora of resources and a legion of supporters, all championing my success. This journey was no longer solely mine; it was our collective odyssey toward hope, healing, and renewal.

8 HEALING THROUGH RELEASE: THE LIBERATING POWER OF FORGIVENESS

~ The Power of Forgiveness~

There's an old keepsake box I've kept for years, hidden away in the back of my closet. Inside, among various trinkets and memories, lies a letter—one I never sent but often read. It's a letter of forgiveness, written in a moment of profound clarity and catharsis. It's addressed to someone who once hurt me deeply, but over the years, the letter became less about them and more about me. It became a symbol of my journey to find peace, release, and healing.

Forgiveness, I've come to realize, is a gift we give ourselves. It's the balm that soothes the raw wounds of betrayal, disappointment, and heartache. Yet, understanding the importance of forgiveness and truly embodying it are two different terrains. The path to forgiving someone, especially when the hurt runs deep, can be winding and steep. And sometimes, the hardest person to forgive is ourselves.

In this chapter, we will embark on a deeply personal exploration of forgiveness. Through my own stories of hurt, reflection, and eventual reconciliation, we'll uncover the transformative power of letting go of past grievances. Together, we'll navigate the complex emotions associated with betrayal and disappointment, seeking to understand how forgiveness can free us from the chains of resentment and bitterness.

As we journey through these pages, you'll find practical strategies, heartfelt reflections, and relatable anecdotes that illuminate the path to forgiveness. This chapter isn't just about understanding the concept of forgiveness—it's an invitation to experience its liberating and healing power firsthand.

I invite you to join me in this intimate voyage as we rediscover the strength, peace, and growth that arises from the act of forgiving. Whether you're seeking to forgive someone else or striving to forgive yourself, remember within forgiveness lies the key to a heart unburdened and a future unshackled.

~My Personal Journey to Forgiving Those Who Hurt Me~

The luminous rays of dawn breaking through the dense curtain of night are often a metaphorical symbol of joy, relief, and liberation. The Bible speaks of it, saying, "Weeping may stay for the night, but rejoicing comes in the morning" (Psalm 30:5). But what if the night seems endless? What if the wounds are so deep that dawn appears unreachable? My journey of forgiveness was my voyage through this elongated night, searching for my morning.

Forgiving those who had scarred my heart was perhaps one of the most intricate mazes I had to navigate. Contrary to popular belief, forgiveness wasn't a single defining moment of magnanimity. It was, for me, a succession of choices, moments of faltering, and retraced steps.

In the initial phase, the very idea of pardoning those who inflicted pain upon me felt counterintuitive. Was I supposed to just overlook the torment? Pretend it never happened? And then it struck me: Forgiveness was not for the transgressors but for the wounded, for me. It was a release from a self-imposed prison where memories of hurt, betrayal, and anguish were my only cellmates.

As days turned to weeks and weeks to months, I slowly recognized that my anger, resentment, and bitterness were not serving me. They were chains binding me to the same individuals and situations I wished to forget. Every time I relived those memories, I gave a piece of my peace to them. It was then I realized that to truly move forward, I had to let go. But how?

Diving deep into my faith and spiritual practices, I began to dissect the layers of my emotions. I sought to understand the perspective of those who wronged me. This didn't mean justifying their actions but attempting to see them as fallible humans, prone to errors, much like myself.

A pivotal point in my journey was meditating upon the scripture about joy coming in the morning. But my "morning" wasn't just the next sunrise; it was the eventual breakthrough after the most extended and darkest hours of my soul. It took days, weeks, years even, for my internal skies to light up with the first rays of understanding, acceptance, and ultimately, forgiveness.

As I embraced this newfound perspective, a weight I hadn't fully realized I was carrying began to lift. The shadows of past grudges started to recede, making way for light, love, and an inner peace I hadn't felt in a long time. By releasing my captors, I had unknowingly set myself free.

In the end, forgiveness was my dawn, my morning filled with joy. And as I reveled in its warmth, I understood that my night, however prolonged, was essential for the appreciation of the coming day.

~Forgiving Oneself: The Path to Inner Peace~

Stepping out from the darkness of forgiving others, a deeper, more complex challenge awaited me: self-forgiveness. Although I had navigated the tough landscape of comprehending and forgiving others, it was glaringly obvious that the journey toward forgiving myself was fraught with its own set of struggles.

Often, our harshest critic lies within. The whispers of our missteps grow louder in the quiet recesses of our minds. For every time I had faltered, betrayed, or disappointed, an echoing voice inside me was there to keep score. Each mistake became an indelible mark, a reminder of my imperfections. The continuous reel of negative self-talk had eroded my self-worth so deeply that I began to perceive myself through the distorted lens of my past errors.

Every stumble in my life was played in a loop, a relentless highlight reel of how I had failed, how I had let others and myself down. Amid this tumultuous internal storm, the lyrics of a song that spoke of rebuilding oneself resonated with me. It became an anthem, an inspiration, guiding me out of my self-inflicted darkness. "Rebuild" by J. Moss became more than just a song; it turned into my silent plea, a prayer, a hope.

To heal and find my way back to my true essence, I had to first understand the depths of my wounds. Recognizing that the harshest judgments I believed were from the world outside were echoing loudest from within me was a revelation. It made me question: Why was I so unkind to myself? Why did I not grant myself the same understanding and grace I offered to others?

In my quest for self-forgiveness, I had to relearn self-love. It started with silencing the insidious voice of self-doubt and shifting the narrative. Instead of fixating on my blunders, I began focusing on my growth, the lessons learned, and the strengths I had forged in the furnace of my past. I started embracing the idea that imperfections are not shortcomings but unique facets that make me who I am.

I repeated affirmations to myself like a mantra, whispering words of encouragement, love, and acceptance. "I am enough. I am worth it." With each repetition it sunk deeper, repairing the cracks in my self-esteem and self-worth.

Forgiving myself was not a single act but a continuous journey. After navigating the turbulent waters of forgiving others, turning inward was like reaching the shores of an uncharted island—intimidating yet promising untapped treasures. It was in this exploration that I unearthed the gem of self-worth.

In understanding and accepting myself, flaws and all, I discovered that inner peace wasn't a destination but a journey. A journey that required constant reflection, learning, and, above all, an undying commitment to self-love and acceptance. It's in this commitment to self that I found my path to genuine inner peace. And the journey continues...

~Strategies and Exercises to Foster Forgiveness~

Embarking on the journey of forgiveness can feel like navigating uncharted waters. The weight of hurt, resentment, and past pain can sometimes feel overwhelming, demanding every ounce of courage and determination to traverse. My path to forgiveness, although laden with challenges, brought profound understanding and peace. This transformative journey is reminiscent of many stories in religious traditions, but one stands out remarkably—the life of Jesus.

Jesus, in His time on Earth, showcased unconditional love and forgiveness in unparalleled ways. Perhaps the most profound act of forgiveness was when He was crucified. Despite enduring unimaginable pain and betrayal, He beseeched, "Father, forgive them, for they do not know what they are doing." In this spirit of boundless forgiveness and compassion, there is a lesson for us all. Through Jesus's example, we can glean the true essence of forgiveness and apply it in our lives.

Drawing from the teachings of Jesus and my own journey, here are strategies and exercises to foster forgiveness:

Compassion Exercise

Jesus was the embodiment of compassion. Reflect on times when you were shown undeserved kindness or mercy. Try to extend that same compassion to those who have wronged you, understanding that every individual has their struggles.

Write a Forgiveness Prayer

Pen down a prayer that specifically focuses on your intent to forgive. Express your feelings and hurt, and ask for the strength to forgive. This act, even if done in private, is a step towards emotional liberation.

Meditative Contemplation

Dedicate quiet moments to reflect on Jesus's teachings about forgiveness. This can be done through scripture reading, meditation, or simple contemplation. Absorb the serenity and strength these teachings provide.

Affirmations of Release

Daily, recite affirmations that resonate with forgiveness and grace. Phrases like "I choose to forgive as I am forgiven" can serve as powerful reminders.

Seek Spiritual Support

Sharing your journey with a spiritual mentor, pastor, or trusted members of your community can be beneficial. Their insights and support can often provide clarity and guidance.

In emulating Jesus's teachings, we learn that forgiveness isn't just about letting go of past grievances but is also a path to profound spiritual growth and inner tranquility. It's a recognition that in offering forgiveness, we free not only the others, more importantly, ourselves.

9 PILLARS OF PROGRESS: CELEBRATING SMALL WINS AND CHERISHING LESSONS

~ The Pillars of Progress: Small Victories, Support, and Lessons Learned

Have you ever found yourself enveloped in darkness, with just a glimmer of light at a distance serving as your only guide? That distant light, though faint, becomes our beacon of hope, urging us forward with the reassurance that the end of darkness is near and a brighter, more hopeful world lies ahead. Our journey through life, marked by numerous challenges and transitions, often resembles that very tunnel. Yet, no matter how suffocating the darkness may seem, there is always that promise of light—a symbol of hope, resilience, and the incredible strength of the human spirit.

In this chapter, we will journey towards that light together. We will delve into the importance of drawing inspiration from small victories, building a support system for seamless transitions, and harnessing the lessons from past transitions for future growth. These are the cornerstones that have not only helped me navigate my own journey but have also empowered countless others to emerge from the darkness into a brighter, more hopeful tomorrow.

Together, we will explore strategies to rekindle hope, even in the face of overwhelming despair. We will delve deep into the transformative power of perseverance, drawing inspiration from those who have navigated challenging paths before us and discovered the light of triumph and renewal on the other side.

As you immerse yourself in this chapter, let it serve as a source of unwavering encouragement. Let each story, each lesson, and each insight empower you to navigate your current challenges with a steadfast belief that brighter days lie ahead.

Embrace this chapter as a rallying cry, a clarion call to never give up, to persistently move forward, no matter how daunting the odds may seem. The light at the end of the tunnel is not just an end to darkness—it is a beginning, a fresh start, a world filled with endless possibilities. Let us journey towards it with conviction, passion, and unrelenting hope.

~Drawing Inspiration from Small Victories~

As I reflect on my journey, I am reminded that while monumental events have brought me immense joy, sometimes the small victories are just as precious, if not more so. The opportunity to wake up each morning feeling alive and ready to face the day is a blessing I do not take for granted. The ability to smile and laugh again after periods of struggle and sorrow is a testament to the resilience of the human spirit. Most importantly, the awareness that God has been by my side through it all, guiding me and supporting me, fills my heart with gratitude and awe.

I have been through so much, faced numerous challenges, and endured my fair share of pain. But now, I feel a sense of renewal. It's my time to shine. Completing this book is a significant milestone for me, one that symbolizes not only the culmination of months of hard work but also my commitment to growth and self-improvement. It's a small victory that holds profound meaning.

In addition to finishing the book, I have been the recipient of random acts of kindness, which have warmed my heart and reminded me of the goodness that exists in the world. Simple gestures, like a stranger holding the door open for me or a friend sending an unexpected message of encouragement, have lifted my spirits and inspired me to pay it forward.

Drawing inspiration from these small victories has been crucial for my well-being and personal development. They serve as reminders that progress is not always measured by grand achievements or significant milestones. Sometimes, it's the little things that make the biggest difference. The daily acts of kindness, the moments of self-care, and the small steps forward collectively contribute to a happier, healthier, and more fulfilling life.

As I move forward, I am committed to celebrating the small victories, both in my own life and in the lives of others. I will continue to find inspiration in the everyday moments that bring joy and contentment. And, with a grateful heart, I will acknowledge the presence of God in my life, trusting that He will continue to guide me and bless me with small victories along the way.

~Building a Support System: Pillars of Strength Through Transitions~

Navigating through life's transitions is never an easy task. Each stage and change comes with its own set of triumphs and trials. Amidst all these continuous evolutions, one thing remains constant and profoundly impactful – the support system that surrounds us. This system, founded on trust, love, and shared experiences, has been my rock, my safe haven, and guiding light through every twist and turn.

My parents have been unwavering in their support and belief in me, standing as the bedrock of encouragement, especially during times when self-doubt clouded my vision. They have been the impetus that drives me onward, igniting a determination within me to surpass my limits.

My sons, the embodiments of my pride and joy, are the anchors in my life, providing a sense of balance and perspective. Their unconditional love and trust are the forces that spur me to strive continually towards being the best version of myself, nurturing in me a sense of purpose and fulfillment.

Solomon, a pillar of strength in my life, plays an indispensable role. He is the compass that guides me towards truth and accountability. With a gentle yet firm hand, Solomon ensures that I stay true to my values and responsibilities. His presence in my life is a constant reminder of the importance of integrity and sincerity. In his unique way, Solomon contributes significantly to my personal growth, challenging me to introspect and evolve continually. His influence is subtle yet profound, fostering in me a deeper understanding of myself and the world around me.

My sisters, from other misters and my brothers, from other mothers, are always there to speak life into me. They laugh with me, shed tears with me, and accept me for who I am, flaws and all. With them, I don't have to pretend to have it all together. They always find a way to break down my hard exterior, knowing that underneath is a soft shell.

One vital part of my support system is Pastor Natasha Rockmore. Her deep reservoir of spiritual wisdom has been a steadfast anchor for me. Our cherished conversations, where scriptures intertwine seamlessly with real-life situations, often offer clarity amidst confusion. Her words, always rooted in faith and kindness, remind me of the bigger picture and the divine play at work.

Another pillar of strength is Apostle Kimberly Jones, my mentor, a spiritual powerhouse. Her insights, deeply rooted in faith, have guided me through many crossroads in life. The lessons she has imparted, both through her words and her own life, have served as a compass, helping me navigate my journey with grace, strength, and purpose.

I pray that each and every one of you find a support system, be it family or friends. I've learned that I can't go it alone. The enemy wants you to be separated, but there is strength in partnerships. Life is a journey filled with continuous change, and having a solid support system is crucial for navigating these transitions. They are the foundation that keeps us steady, the refuge that offers comfort, and the guiding light that directs us through the darkness. Together, we can overcome any obstacle and emerge stronger on the other side.

~ Harnessing the Lessons from Past Transitions for Future Growth~

Our journey through existence is anything but a straight road filled with predictable events. It guides us through valleys, escorts us up mountains, and sometimes plunges us into the churning waters of change. Moments of transition, regardless of their size, harbor potent lessons that subsequently direct our future adventures. By accepting these transitions and the wisdom they bestow, we do more than just survive; we prosper, evolving into stronger, wiser, and more resilient beings.

My journey is a testament to the transformative power of transitions. Reflecting on the many changes I've navigated; I've realized that each one was a hidden classroom. There were moments when the lessons were harsh, requiring grit and resilience. Other times, they were gentle reminders of my own strength and potential. Regardless of their nature, they have collectively shaped me into who I am today.

One crucial lesson transitions have taught me is the art of perseverance. The ability to push forward, even when the path is filled with obstacles, has been a cornerstone of my growth.

With each hurdle I've faced, I've realized that the challenges aren't permanent fixtures but mere stepping stones, each one leading to a brighter horizon.

Another essential takeaway has been the understanding that healing is a layered process. Every hurt, no matter how deep or scalding, has the potential to be mended. But it requires time, patience, and, often, the loving support of those around us. Just as a wound doesn't heal overnight, emotional and mental healing has its own timeline. Acknowledging this has allowed me to give myself the grace to recover at my own pace.

Furthermore, transitions have highlighted the importance of adaptability. Life is a dynamic entity, constantly evolving and shifting. By learning to adapt and evolve with it, I've not only managed to ride the waves of change but have also found joy and growth in the process.

Lastly, and perhaps most profoundly, these periods of change have underscored the importance of self-belief. Believing in my own potential, even when external voices were skeptical, has been my guiding light. It has fueled my spirit to conquer challenges, heal from adversities, and continuously strive towards becoming the best version of myself.

As I stand today, looking back at the woven narrative of my life, I am filled with gratitude for every twist and turn. Each transition, with its unique set of lessons, has been instrumental in shaping me. As the saying goes, "What doesn't break you makes you stronger." I am living proof of that. With the wisdom of the past firmly in my grasp, I am poised and ready for whatever the future holds, knowing that each new transition will only add another chapter to my ever-evolving story of growth and rebirth.

As Proverbs 3:5-6 says, "Trust in the Lord with all your heart and lean not on your own understanding; in all your ways submit to him, and he will make your paths straight." This scripture has been a constant reminder for me to trust in a higher power during times of transition and change. It reassures me that even when the path seems uncertain, there is a greater plan at work, guiding me toward my true purpose.

10 LIFE'S ETERNAL DANCE: EMBRACING THE CONTINUAL RHYTHMS OF CHANGE

~ The Constant of Change~

Years ago, while leafing through an old family album, I stumbled upon a photograph of myself as a child. That bright-eyed, carefree girl seemed worlds away from the woman I had become. Yet, as I traced the journey from that moment captured in time to the present, I was struck by the one undeniable constant: change. The seasons in the background had shifted, the surroundings had transformed, and the young girl had evolved, each transition marking a distinct chapter of life.

Life, in all its magnificent unpredictability, is a tapestry of changes. From the monumental shifts to the subtle everyday evolutions, change is the thread that weaves our stories, shaping our identities, aspirations, and dreams. It's both the challenge we grapple with and the force that propels us forward.

In this concluding chapter, we will reflect upon the journey we've undertaken together through the pages of this book.

Revisiting the insights, lessons, and moments of revelation, we'll celebrate the resilience and growth that come hand-in-hand with embracing life's transitions. Drawing from my own experiences and the shared wisdom of countless souls who've traversed similar paths, we'll ponder the beautiful, unending cycle of life and renewal.

As we wrap up this journey, let this chapter be a gentle reminder that while change is inevitable, our response to it is a choice. The stories, strategies, and reflections shared within these pages aim to guide, but it's your personal narrative, your unique journey, which breathes life into them.

Join me in this final reflection as we embrace the ever-present constant of change, cherishing the memories, lessons, and hopes it brings along. And as we close this chapter, let's step forward with a heart full of gratitude, wisdom, and anticipation for the myriad transitions yet to come.

~Embracing Change as a Part of Our Human Journey~

Transformation, in its various manifestations, is a guaranteed element of our human voyage. At the heart of every pulse, the soul of every exhale, and the base of every aspiration lies the undertow of transformation. Although it is so fundamental to our being, it often feels like a turbulent tempest, unsettling our souls and casting clouds of skepticism on our routes. In these moments of doubt, I have discovered that relying on a steadfast faith in God becomes our guiding star, steering us through the storm and into tranquility.

In retrospect, I can perceive God's influence in coordinating each transition I have encountered. Whether it was a door that shut, only for a window to emerge, or a hurdle that seemed impossible at the moment, His presence was a constant. These transitions, regardless of how disconcerting they felt at the time, were divinely designated stepping stones, assisting me in climbing to elevated perspectives of comprehension, empathy, and purpose.

Nothing we face in our journey is mere coincidence. The twists and bends, the joys and sorrows, the triumphs and setbacks—each is a segment in our distinct narrative, meticulously composed by God. And while it is human instinct to oppose or even dread change, welcoming it with faith enables us to recognize it for what it truly is: an opportunity. An opportunity to develop, transform, and approach the divine blueprint God has for each of us.

The scripture states, "For I know the plans I have for you, declares the Lord, plans for welfare and not for evil, to give you a future and a hope." This vow, this heavenly guarantee, is a testament to the fact that even when our world appears to be shifting beneath our feet, there is a superior plan in motion. A plan that is founded in love, purpose, and an unwavering belief in our potential.

As I have maneuvered through the various transitions in my life, from the most trivial to the most revolutionary, I have realized that trust is the compass that guides us correctly. Trust in God's timing, trust in His wisdom, and trust in the journey He has mapped out for us. Even when the path is unclear, when the next step appears intimidating, this trust is what grants us the bravery to progress.

Fundamentally, change is not merely a component of our human journey; it is its very essence. It is the crucible where our character is shaped, our faith is examined, and our spirits are elevated. And with God as our anchor, each transition, each moment of change, becomes a portal to unmatched growth, leading us to the next glorious chapter of our lives. As we accept change, we accept the limitless possibilities God has embedded in our path, knowing that with Him by our side, the journey is as beautiful as the destination.

~The Divine Blueprint: Rediscovering Myself in Christ~

For years, the person I truly was remained hidden beneath layers of hurt, doubt, shame, and unforgiveness that I carried around like a heavyweight. I felt broken, used, and abused. Who could possibly love me in all my brokenness? My identity crisis was further exacerbated by the fact that my biological mother is part of the LGBTQ community. As a child and teen, I didn't know how to process that. It made me homophobic for years, and it made me question my own womanhood and identity.

I constantly compared myself to others, convinced they were somehow better than me. This led to deep dissatisfaction with myself, and for many years, I couldn't bear the person staring back at me in the mirror. I was Dawn Love, but I struggled to accept and embrace that identity. Instead, I tried to morph myself into what others expected or wanted me to be, shrinking myself to fit into molds that were not meant for me.

This journey was tiresome and soul-draining, keeping me disconnected from my true self. It wasn't until I turned to Christ that I began to understand the depth of my identity crisis. The Bible offered a powerful and transformative truth: "Therefore, if anyone is in Christ, he is a new creation. The old has passed away; behold, the new has come" (2 Corinthians 5:17). This verse became a pivotal point in my journey of self-discovery.

My quest to uncover my identity in Christ resembled a spiritual excavation. With each scripture, prayer, and moment of reflection, I peeled away the layers of insecurity, doubt, and fear that had obscured my true self. I began to understand that I was intricately designed by God, a masterpiece in His eyes. My value was not determined by worldly judgments, past failures, or the accolades I had accumulated. Instead, my worth was rooted in the undeniable truth that I was created in the image of the Divine, a beloved child of God.

Accepting this revelation was transformative. It changed not only how I perceived myself but also how I interacted with the world. I started to love the person I was becoming and found joy in the smallest moments and purpose in the challenges I faced. My actions, fueled by a renewed sense of self-awareness and acceptance, became more aligned with God's will. The void created by my identity crisis was filled with a passion to live as Christ intended, embodying His love, grace, and purpose.

Today, you will encounter a new Dawn. I am the one with a loud voice, a contagious laugh, and a heart that loves deeply. I am unapologetically myself, and I love the person I have become.

I am God's blueprint, crafted in His image and empowered to fulfill my divine purpose. My journey to self-awareness, acceptance, and action was intimately linked to my relationship with Christ. By grounding my identity in Him, I found the freedom to be my most authentic self. A life once dominated by doubt has been transformed into one marked by conviction and purpose. I no longer thrive on the world's standards but on the profound truth of who I am in Christ: cherished, worthy, and empowered.

~A Final Word: The Unending Cycle of Life and Renewal~

As I sit here, fingers poised over the keyboard, reflecting on the words and stories I've woven throughout this book, a profound sense of gratitude washes over me. It's a gratitude grounded in the recognition that the seeds of this journey were sown by a power much greater than my own. The gentle hand of God planted the very essence of this book deep within my soul. And with divine patience, He watered and pruned, crafting every chapter and every line, guiding me through moments of doubt, and lifting me during moments of inspiration.

I have come to realize that transitions are sacred. They are the profound markers of the unending cycle of life and renewal. They've taken me on a journey from the depths of despair to the peaks of joy. With each transition, a layer of the old me is shed away, revealing a version closer to the woman God envisioned. A version stronger, wiser, more compassionate, and infinitely more in tune with the divine.

It's easy for many to look back at transitions with regret or resentment, focusing solely on the pain they caused. But I've learned to see them as blessings, as essential milestones on my journey of growth and self-discovery. It's through these transitions, these moments of profound change, that I've been reborn time and time again, evolving into a woman deeply rooted in faith, fortified by experience, and radiant with God's love.

Without these transitions, without these pivotal moments of transformation, I wouldn't be the woman I am today. There were times I felt lost in the wilderness, times I grappled with my identity and purpose. Yet, it was during these challenging times I forged my strength and resilience. It took sweat, tears, and unyielding faith to become this woman. I fought battles both external and internal. I wrestled with demons of doubt, fear, and insecurity. But with God by my side, guiding me through every storm, I emerged victorious. I fought like hell to become her, and now, I wear my scars with pride, a testament to my journey and God's unwavering grace.

Knowing who I am today, I can say with unwavering confidence, "I AM UNSTOPPABLE." The journey may not have been easy, and I anticipate more transitions on the horizon, for the story is far from over. But with God as my guide, I'm ready to embrace whatever lies ahead with open arms and an unwavering spirit.

With this final reflection, I want to leave you with a message of hope, resilience, and self-acceptance. Know that it's okay to celebrate yourself, to encourage yourself, and to be your own cheerleader. Your journey, with all its challenges and victories, is shaping you into the person you are meant to be. Embrace it with open arms and a grateful heart. And always, always remember with faith, with trust in God's plan, and with a steadfast commitment to your own growth, YOU ARE RELENTLESS.

As this chapter closes and the book draws to its end, remember this: Life's transitions are not roadblocks; they're stepping stones, guiding you toward the person you are destined to become. There are still many pages to fill, many adventures to embark on, and many lessons to learn. Cherish them, learn from them, and always, always move forward with faith.

To God be the glory, forever and ever. Amen

PRAYER GUIDE:
NAVIGATING TRANSITIONS

Understanding Transitions

Heavenly Father, grant me the wisdom to recognize the seasons of change, the serenity to accept them, and the understanding to discern their deeper meanings. As I face the inevitable flow of life, let my heart remain anchored in Your constant love.

Vulnerability as Strength

Dear Lord, in moments of vulnerability, remind me of the strength I found in surrender. Teach me to open my heart to Your guiding hand, knowing that, in my raw authenticity, I find true power and connection.

Challenges as Stepping stones

Almighty God, when challenges arise, help me see them not as obstacles but as steppingstones. Strengthen my resolve, that I may face adversity with courage, knowing each trial is but a lesson in Your grand design.

Finding God Amidst the Storm

In the midst of life's tempests, O Lord, be my refuge. Even when the path is unclear, let Your presence be the light that guides me, reminding me that even the fiercest storm is under Your sovereign command.

The Pillars of Resilience and Fortitude

God of all comfort, fortify my spirit. In times of upheaval, instill in me a resilience that reflects Your enduring love, and grant me the fortitude to stand firm in faith, even when the ground beneath shakes.

Navigating Emotional Upheavals

Gracious God, when emotions surge and ebb, grant me the grace to navigate them with wisdom. Let my heart find solace in Your eternal truths and, in moments of emotional tumult, remind me of Your unchanging love.

Rebuilding After Setbacks

Master Builder, when life breaks me down, inspire me to rebuild with You as my foundation. Let each setback be a steppingstone to a stronger, more resilient self, always rooted in Your purpose.

The Power of Forgiveness

Lord of Mercy, teach me the art of forgiveness. Soften my heart towards those who've hurt me and guide me in the journey of healing. As I seek to forgive, let me never forget the boundless forgiveness You bestow upon me daily.

The Light at the End of the Tunnel

O God, my guiding light, in the darkest of times, shine Your radiant hope upon my path. Let me always move towards Your brilliance, seeking the warmth of Your love and the promise of a new dawn.

Navigating Life's Transitions: A Comprehensive Toolkit

My God, arm me with the tools to journey through life's transitions with grace and poise. Bless me with discernment, resilience, and unwavering faith, ensuring every step I take is aligned with Your divine plan.

The Constant of Change

Eternal God, in the ever-changing landscape of life, You remain my unchanging rock. As I embrace the twists and turns of my journey, let my heart always find rest in Your immutable truths and steadfast love.

****

May these prayers serve as a beacon of light and comfort, guiding and strengthening you as you navigate the transitions of life. Remember: in every change, God's unchanging hand is always there to guide, protect, and bless you.

THANK YOU!

Dear Reader,

From the depths of my heart, thank you for choosing to journey through the pages of my book. It is a privilege to share my thoughts and experiences with you, and I genuinely hope they resonated or brought you some comfort or insight. Your support means the world to me. Each reader breathes life into the words I've penned, making the effort and vulnerability of writing truly worthwhile. May you carry forward whatever you've gleaned, and may it serve you well in your own life's journey.

With immense gratitude,

JUST DAWN LOVE

ABOUT THE AUTHOR

Dawn Love, the heart and soul behind JUST DAWN LOVE, LLC, is a beacon of inspiration in myriad roles – from a passionate Minister to an adept CEO. At the heart of her ministry, Dawn's love for Christ is luminous, epitomized by her favorite scripture: "With God, all things are possible." This fervor translates seamlessly into her teachings, illuminating minds with profound Gospel insights through her Bible studies.

Possessing a BS in Psychology and an MA in Human Services, Dawn's academic prowess harmoniously merges with her spiritual calling. Specializing in life coaching, she's pioneered the transformative coaching service, "Transition with Love," under the God-ordained platform "Transitions." This venture serves as a beacon, helping individuals traverse life's significant shifts and adapt with grace and resilience.

As a mentor, Dawn's touchstone is guiding young women, offering solace and direction during life's challenging phases. Her voice, both inspirational and motivational, has echoed far and wide, not just through personal interactions but also via her Facebook Live show, "Live to Inspire." Here, she showcases indomitable spirits who've mastered life's transitions, offering hope and encouragement to countless souls.

Dawn's commitment to serve, encourage, motivate, and inspire is evident in every endeavor she undertakes. It's a reflection of her deep-rooted desire to uplift others to their highest potential.

Beyond her professional accolades, Dawn is a doting mother to three beautiful souls and has planted her roots in the vibrant Atlanta area. Dive deeper into her world by visiting www.justdawnlove.com.

In the symphony of life, where Dawn orchestrates multiple roles with poise and grace when the music fades, she remains, at her very essence, Just Dawn Love. A relatable soul, exuding genuine power and authenticity.

www.ingramcontent.com/pod-product-compliance
Lightning Source LLC
Chambersburg PA
CBHW052215270326
41931CB00011B/2357